Superior Productivity
in Health Care Organizations

Superior Productivity
in Health Care Organizations

How to Get It,
How to Keep It

by
Paul Fogel, M.B.A.
Executive Information Systems, Inc.

**HEALTH
PROFESSIONS
PRESS**

Baltimore • London • Winnipeg • Sydney

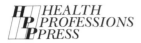

HEALTH PROFESSIONS PRESS

Health Professions Press, Inc.
Post Office Box 10624
Baltimore, Maryland 21285-0624

www.healthpropress.com

Typeset by Barton Matheson Willse & Worthington, Baltimore, Maryland.
Manufactured in the United States of America by
Versa Press, East Peoria, Illinois.

All of the case studies in this book are composites of the author's actual
experiences. In all instances, names have been changed; in some instances,
identifying details have been altered to further protect confidentiality.

All financial data in this book are fictional and are provided only for illustrative
purposes to demonstrate typical financial and business practices.

Library of Congress Cataloging-in-Publication Data
Fogel, Paul (Paul Allan), 1958–
    Superior productivity in health care organizations/by Paul Fogel.
        p.   cm.
    Includes index.
    ISBN 1-87881-293-9
    1. Health facilities—Personnel management.   2. Health facilities—Labor
productivity.   3. Health services administration.   I. Title.
    RA971.35.F64   2003
    362.11/0683 22   2003056732

British Library Cataloguing in Publication data are available from the British Library.

C • O • N • T • E • N • T • S

About the Author ix
Preface xi
Introduction xvii

Chapter 1 The State of the Union 1
Been There, Done That 2
Do Layoffs Really Work? 4
Skill Mix Strategy . . . . : 6
Benchmarking 10
Problem of Overtime and Registry 13
   Sample Overtime and Registry Analysis 15
   Strategies for Reducing Overtime and Registry 17
   Float Pools 19
Hospital Mergers 20
   Market-Based Solution 22
Summary 23

Chapter 2 How to Develop Realistic Productivity
           Standards 27
Learn From History 27
Assign Performance Measures 28
   Performance Measures for the Entire Organization 30
Do the Math 32
   How to Prepare the Analysis 33
   Illustration: 3-Year Productivity Analysis 33
   Don't Forget Registry 36
   Float Pool 37
   Communicating the Findings 37
   How Many Years Are Best for the Analysis? 48
   What to Expect 49
After the Analysis 50
   Translating the Analysis into Standards 51
   There Are No Shortcuts 53
Do You Need Outside Help? 54
   Executive Commitment 55

How Long Will This Take? 55
Managing for Change 56
Comparing Apples and Oranges 58
Illustration: Accounting for Changing Service or Patient Mix . . .59
Internal Benchmarking 61
Summary 62

Chapter 3   Implementation 65
Fixed and Variable: Fact or Fiction? 66
Mechanics of Fixed/Variable Splitting 67
Fixed and Variable within the Department 68
Illustration 69
Don't Shield Managers from Managing 72
The New Deal 73
Let Managers Manage 73
Don't Take Testimony 74
Budget Discipline—Missing in Action 75
Accountability: The Brave New World 78
Individual Accountability 78
Executive Accountability 81
Terms of the Deal 84
Implications for Managers 85
What Is in it for Us? 86
Rules for Changing Standards 89
The New Deal: Harsh or Kind? 93
Implementation Strategy 95
Relate Productivity to Strategic Goals 95
Allow for a Transition Period 96
How Long Should the Transition Take? 98
Factor in the Composition of Labor 99
Summary 101

Chapter 4   Monitoring and Reporting 105
Seduced by Technology 105
Technology and Good Management .105
Complex Systems Do Not Work 108
The Law of Unintended Consequences 108
Timing of Reviews 110
Reporting Frequency 112
The New Productivity Report 113
How to Create Your Own Report 115

Format of the Productivity Report 116
How to Analyze the Report 117
Make the Master Schedule Work 120
Adjusting Staffing Schedules 122
Guidelines for Fixed Departments 123
Summary 124

Chapter 5   Incentives and Consequences 127
Laying the Foundation 128
Incentives 130
End Symbolic Efforts 131
Why Should We Change? .133
Quality Standards 134
How to Draft an Effective Incentive Plan 137
Executive Incentives 138
Manager Incentives 142
Consequences 148
How to Draft an Effective Productivity Policy 152
Six Principles of an Effective Productivity Policy 153
Establishing the Proper Limits 154
Keep It Public 155
Productivity Committee Procedure 156
Parting Company 157
Summary *158*

Chapter 6   The Politics of Productivity 161
Medical Staff 162
Labor Unions 164
Executives 166
Department Managers 167
The Board 168
Productivity for the Long Term 169
Summary 170

Appendix   Case Studies 173
Emergency Room 173
Dietary 176
Mother/Baby Unit 178

Glossary of Terms 181
Index 185

A•B•O•U•T T•H•E A•U•T•H•O•R

Paul Fogel is the President of Executive Information Systems, Inc. The firm produces a financial reporting and forecasting system for hospitals and offers services in productivity improvement, benchmarking, operations analysis, feasibility studies, and business planning. Mr. Fogel offers a unique perspective gained from working in more than 50 hospitals.

Mr. Fogel wrote the feature article for the August 2000 issue of *Healthcare Financial Management* magazine titled "Achieving Superior Productivity." The Healthcare Financial Management Association (HFMA) also hired him to conduct a workshop called "Benchmarking in Action."

After earning an MBA, Mr. Fogel began work as a financial analyst with several commercial and savings banks and later moved on to venture capital, and then to hospitals as Manager of Strategic Business Analysis, reporting to the CFO. In 1995, he joined MECON, Inc., a national benchmarking and consulting firm to the health care industry (later a division of GE Medical Systems). As senior manager, he educated, trained, and consulted with more than 40 different hospitals, including the United States Army. Becoming self-employed in 1997, Mr. Fogel engaged in extensive long-term work with a Seattle hospital as a productivity and benchmarking consultant. In 1999, he concluded an engagement with the fourteen hospitals of California's Catholic Healthcare West chain. In 2003, he completed work on a financial reporting, productivity, and budgeting system for hospitals and formed a company to bring it to market.

P • R • E • F • A • C • E

Productivity management, central as it is to financial health, is a mysterious topic to most administrators and department managers. Not having a body of literature that clearly points the way to what works in the real world is partly to blame. Industry journals address the subject in piecemeal fashion, and such literature is accessible only to a specialized audience. In fact, as of 2003 there is no other book on hospital productivity management currently in print. Certainly, there are many general management books, but it is difficult to know how to apply them specifically to the hospital industry.

From my perspective as a professional consultant in productivity improvement, benchmarking, operations analysis, forecasting, and business planning, too often hospitals are buying hopes and dreams, spending time and money on purely temporary gains. Cut first and ask questions later? Ask yourself this: Will we have to do this all over again in a year or two?

Of course, many consulting firms do good analytical work, but their approach often lacks a conceptual framework that fits productivity into the overall management structure of the hospital. The conventional approach leaves intact the existing management configuration with all of its policies and procedures. If existing management practices remain untouched, if the same things are tried again, then the same results will be repeated. If health care organizations are not happy with the previous results, they will not be any happier this time. That is not the approach taken by this book. This book is a practical guide to achieving superior productivity at any organization that is willing to take on the challenge. Moreover, such fundamental change can be done at a fraction of the cost and time that consulting firms might charge.

It is too easy to blame an indifferent Congress, wicked HMOs, greedy labor unions, tight labor markets, overregulation, and a million other things over which managers have essentially no control. No doubt, these pose serious challenges. Troubled organizations could be pushed over the edge into bankruptcy. However, there is much under management control. It is all very well to manage an organization in prosperous times. The real test comes when faced with challenges that threaten existence, those that demand fundamental changes in how business is conducted. Many other industries are heavily regulated—airlines, construction, and banking, to name a few. Yet, excellent management finds a way to eke out a profit regardless. They learn, they adapt, they experiment, and they survive. Health care can do the same. If hospitals fail as an enterprise, it will be largely of their own making.

Many organizations may not survive these challenges. They will be merged, bought up, or closed. The survivors will distinguish themselves by challenging entrenched policy and procedure that worked well in another time, but are failing today, and replacing these with the business ethic of entrepreneurship and innovation, injecting fresh vigor into their organizations. The goal cannot be merely to survive, limping along for one more year.

In this book, I identify the central issue as management responsibility and accountability. The two terms are not identical but are complementary. This means the focus is not on technology and monitoring software but on management structures that address consequences for poor management, incentives for achieving superior outcomes, and a process that drives responsibility and accountability down to the proper management level. No amount of software or "budget policing" can make up for a lack of individual responsibility and accountability. The core issue has always been, and always will be, management.

This book focuses on explaining the underlying management philosophy necessary for developing superior productivity. Based on my experience with more than 50 hospitals, detailed implementation plans without any concepts behind them are destined to fail. The reality is that we cannot design or execute our implementation plans flawlessly. Unforeseen events crop up that must be dealt with. If the implementation team is well versed on the underlying management concepts, then they will be equipped to deal with any snags that may arise. We have to draw the conceptual blueprints before building the house.

Most hospitals have the technical expertise to implement these concepts. The approach of this book is not ruthless, unethical, or disjointed. All of it is presented as a package, and each component supports the whole program.

Here are some of the problems that hospitals face:

- Profitability is eroding at many health systems. Even while hospitals are becoming filled with patients, many hospitals are encountering profitless growth.
- Conventional organizations generate conventional results. We keep trying the same practices, hoping for better results than what we got last time.
- Central planning no longer works. Top-down micromanagement has serious limitations in a technologically sophisticated industry with an educated workforce.

Here are some of the goals that hospitals try to reach:

- Bring labor costs, the largest expense in the organization, under control. Define what constitutes good management, and create real accountability to achieve that end. Build security and prosperity for the organization by creating a sustainable economic foundation.
- Remove arbitrariness and politics from decisions. Develop superior analytical expertise. Learn to live by certain ground rules and values that everyone can understand and accept.

The challenge of productivity management is how to turn around the operating structure, culture, and prevailing incentives that counteract lasting results. Any program involving significant change runs into this hidden problem, and it is often unrecognized or ignored. Procedure and policy, incentives and disincentives will have to change before we can change behavior. Hospital culture will follow. This book describes how to do that.

My purpose is to help you turn your health care organization into a prosperous and secure organization, the best place in which to work and practice. Is such a thing possible with Medicare, Medicaid, and managed care paying the bills? I think it is. Improvement is always possible. Most hospitals have already reduced management layers and the average length of a hospital stay. Those were the right things to do then. Now it is time for the next wave of performance improvement.

Much of what I propose in this book takes proper time to conceptualize, develop, analyze, fund, execute, and monitor. There are no shortcuts. For those in a hurry, remember that the short-term was the long-term one year ago.

This book is a call to action for hospital administrators, physicians, corporate health system staff, and other people of authority and leadership. They have the power to effect change, but they cannot do it alone. They will need to collaborate with their clinical and technical managers, financial analysts, and consultants.

> FOR EVERY PROBLEM, THERE IS A SIMPLE SOLUTION—AND IT IS USUALLY WRONG.
>
> —H.L. MENCKEN

On a related note, this book represents a management philosophy of fairness, clear expectations, discipline, and rules, although it does not delve into developing the personal skills that make for great managers: working relationships built on trust, mutual respect, and what some call "emotional intelligence." Readers interested in learning more may want to acquire *Becoming an Effective Health Care Manager: The Essential Skills of Leadership*, by Len Sperry, Ph.D. (Health Professions Press, 2003).

Is the program in this book the last word on productivity? No single book can be a complete compendium of everything a health care organization can do. This book will get you off to a fast start, give you the wherewithal to keep it going for the long term, and yield considerable, lasting savings. After that, the potential for further improvement is limitless. If your organization implements the program in this book, I would like to document your results so that others can learn from your experience. I would be delighted to hear your reactions, opinions, and comments. You can reach me by writing to fogel@easystreet.com.

I • N • T • R • O • D • U • C • T • I • O • N

At many hospitals, revenues are not keeping pace with expenses. If patient volume is growing, then additional costs often consume all supplementary revenue. If patient volume is stable, then revenue growth is frequently inadequate to offset rising overhead expenses. Whatever the case may be, expenses must match revenues, or deteriorating margins will jeopardize the organization's mission. The purpose of this book is to help organizations move from weakness to strength by controlling their largest single expense—labor. The book lays out enduring, practical solutions to the continual challenge of improving productivity. This program can be achieved in a surprisingly short time and at low cost.

The first chapter outlines where the industry stands in its current approaches to labor management, including layoffs, changing the skill mix, benchmarking, overtime and registry, and hospital mergers. This book helps readers chart a simple, yet highly effective method for developing superior productivity: Chapter 2 shows how to develop standards, Chapter 3 is concerned with implementation, Chapter 4 addresses monitoring, and Chapter 5 deals with incentives and consequences. Finally, Chapter 6 takes up organization politics. The diagram on page xviii presents each of these chapters as spokes on a wheel with the hub being productivity standards. The appendix presents actual case studies, taking readers through the process, from analysis to implementation and beyond. The glossary of terms provides definitions for all relevant terms appearing in the text.

This book addresses productivity throughout the health care organization, stressing concepts of accountability, measurement, fairness, and simplicity. The program summary beginning on page xviii gives an overview of the method for developing superior productivity as it is presented in the book.

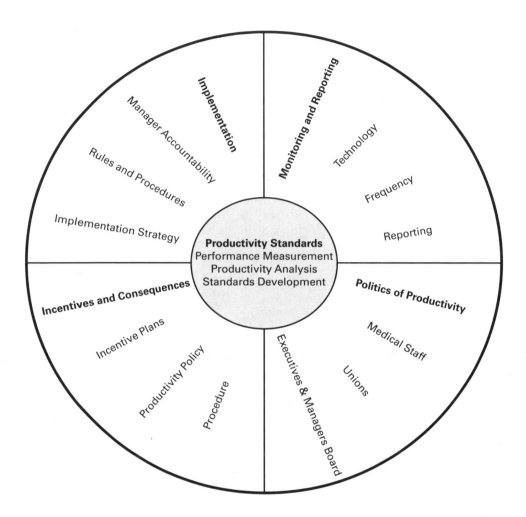

PROGRAM SUMMARY

1. Evaluate each department against its own performance over the last several years. Using history as a standard against which to evaluate current performance is called *historical* benchmarking.

2. Establish monitoring reports and management protocols that executives and managers will follow. These reports and protocols tie directly to the organization's objectives. They are sim-

ple to read and understand, and reflect true underlying trends against which to measure performance. Monitoring can be easy to set up and maintain indefinitely *without* expensive and troublesome software to install, licensing fees, contracts, or multiple year entanglements.

3. Institute a powerful set of incentives and consequences. Managers need clear consequences for poor management. They also need incentives for superior performance. Without these incentives and consequences enshrined in policy, efforts to increase productivity will not work.

Taking into account the hospital's unique culture, traditions, and strategic goals, rules and principles replace politics and the taking of "testimony." The organization will find that it is much easier and more effective to manage by rules and principles than by exception.

The goal is lasting prosperity, not financial turmoil from month to month. To do this, organizations have to allow a high level of autonomy and establish accountability for results so that managers have both the authority and the incentive to pursue what is good for the organization.

THE STATE
OF THE UNION

This introductory chapter is an overview of popular productivity strategies and the reasons why they have come up short. Common strategies to cut labor costs include layoffs, centralization of administrative functions within health care systems, skill mix changes in clinical departments, and controlling overtime and agency use.

All health care systems are concerned with productivity because labor accounts for the bulk of an organization's expenses. Every organization uses some form of productivity measurement system to monitor performance and maintain control of labor costs. As organizations contemplate the purchase of newer, more sophisticated systems, the central question to be answered is this: Why have such systems not reduced costs?

For a variety of reasons, the intent of productivity systems can be easily defeated, setting the stage for severe financial problems down the road. Often unrecognized, but widespread, these reasons must be acknowledged and addressed before organizations can design and implement an effective productivity improvement program that will yield lasting results. Where do productivity programs go wrong? Contributing factors include

- Creation of overly complex measurement and reporting systems
- Failure to establish clear accountability for productivity
- Lack of authority at the appropriate management level
- Short review cycles that highlight temporary or random events
- Lack of incentives to improve and disincentives to prevent decline

BEEN THERE, DONE THAT

Productivity commands constant attention because labor is the largest single expense in service enterprises such as the health care industry. Yet, despite a focus on productivity, every "solution" devised proves to be fleeting. Many organizations go from problem to solution and back again in a circle of frustration. Nothing seems to work for very long.

Despite similar management and organizational structures across the industry, every organization seems to have its own approach to managing productivity—its own policies and procedures, authorities and approvals, and timing and review cycles. Below the surface, however, the way that health care systems actually form their productivity strategies and tactics is strikingly similar:

- *Excessive reliance on the "wisdom" of the budget:* This represents a powerful (if misplaced) desire to adhere to what, in reality, is nothing more than a forecast. Like budgets, almost every forecast is wrong—either too high or too low. Forecasts are valuable for other reasons, but setting productivity standards is not one of them. "Flexible budgets" have been introduced as an improvement over the traditional "fixed" budget. A flexible budget is actually a recalculated budget that takes into account actual workload volumes, not budgeted volumes (i.e., flexible with actual volumes). Using budgeted ratios, expenses are recalculated each month using actual volumes. The resulting flexible budget represents what the budget would have been if the financial planners had perfect knowledge of patient volumes and service mixes while the budget was being drafted. Although the flexible budget is an important advance in budgeting, productivity standards still have to be developed ahead of time to "feed" the budget, whether flexible or fixed.

- *Complex measurement and reporting systems:* Although ostensibly aimed at gaining precise control, complexity confounds the need for simple and clear monitoring, thwarting the ability to act. Management ends up quarreling over numbers instead of getting the results the organization must have.

- *No clear accountability:* Executives are usually in complete control of hiring decisions, setting the number of staff in each department. As a practical necessity, however, executives must delegate accountability to their department managers. Because accountability cannot be delegated without also delegating authority, the result is that no one is truly accountable.

- *Lack of authority at the right level:* Department managers generally have the responsibility for staffing properly or appropriately in their departments, but they usually have little or no hiring power. Without authority where it belongs, blame is created, not accountability.

- *Short review cycles:* Short periods—2 weeks being most typical— serve only to highlight normal statistical variation and obscure meaningful trends. Not really knowing either the problem or the potential of each department, senior management can become paralyzed and feel out of control.

- *No incentives or disincentives:* Once it is able to locate and quantify problems and opportunities, management typically has no meaningful incentives or disincentives to do anything about it.

The lack of incentives and disincentives is probably the top reason why it takes a financial scare to prod many organizations into action. Moreover, such action usually proves to be remarkably short-lived.

• *No shareholder oversight:* With regard to financial performance, nonprofit hospitals (most of the industry) do not have the unity of purpose and the extra measure of oversight that shareholders force on management. Whether the nonprofit, charitable designation is a good thing is beside the point; the fact is that shareholders perform a valuable function for investor-owned hospitals. Nonprofits must find a way to replicate a similar mechanism so that they, too, have the extra discipline such oversight imposes.

DO LAYOFFS REALLY WORK?

Layoffs have been the health care industry's preferred labor cost-control method. Despite this, layoffs have been a colossal failure. For such a desperate and extreme measure, one that greatly disturbs the lives of its victims, it would be reasonable to expect that the tactic at least achieve its objectives. This is far from the case. There are almost never any long-term benefits (more than 2 years) from layoffs.

Across-the-board cuts and layoffs have simply not worked. In a study of 281 cost-cutting campaigns reviewed by consultants E.C. Murphy (1996a), more than 70% of these efforts produced no significant cost savings. Even worse, any initial savings produced by radical cuts virtually disappeared over the next 18–24 months. Although staff can always be eliminated, it is much more difficult to do away with their work. Work processes and tasks remain un-

ACTION	PREDICTABLE RESULT
Unexpected layoffs	Temporary cost cutting, offset by • Severance pay • Outplacement benefits • Extended fringe benefits • Morale problems • Possible flight of highly skilled, most "marketable" employees
Dramatic, wide-spread layoffs	Patient care quality suffers

Figure 1.1. Layoff scorecard.

changed, but with fewer people to do the same work, something usually suffers: Backlogs begin accumulating; the quality of care may deteriorate, and employee morale is hurt, causing productivity declines. In response, staff size gradually increases to former levels. The cycle repeats when the next cost-crunch strikes. Figure 1.1 explains the results of layoffs.

Another study by E.C. Murphy (1996b) linked dramatic across-the-board cuts to mortality. Of 27 hospitals that downsized more than 7.5%, 81% had a "higher mortality rate than predicted." Although the study used a small sample size, it should be enough to give anyone pause.

In almost every case, a layoff (more politely called a *reduction in force*) indicates a lack of foresight and good planning in the face of known economic trends. The preferred course of action is to plan and continually adjust labor resources to work demands so that layoffs are unnecessary. If the organization does not let its labor costs get out of control, periodic crisis adjustments are avoided. If the organization is running out of cash and will soon close its doors, however, there may be no other recourse.

SKILL MIX STRATEGY

Skill mix refers to the average level of training, certification, and experience in departments. By shifting to less-experienced, lower-certified, less-capable employees (e.g., replacing a registered nurse [RN] with a licensed vocational nurse [LVN]), the hope is that the organization can save money. Skill mix changes usually pencil out nicely, making them attractive on paper. It follows that cheaper employees save on labor costs—or do they?

Although *potential* savings can always be found by changing the skill mix to a lower level of employee, problems of supervision, workflow, efficiency, and clinical outcomes often surface. Because of this, in the real world, organizations are seldom able to sustain a one-for-one substitution for any length of time. With the skill mix strategy, organizations have more people, not fewer. That means more supervision, further handoffs, added interruptions, and more benefit plans to administer. In short, the organization must deal with these unforeseen and unintended consequences that never make it into the financial analysis. The literature and real-world experience demonstrate that the best productivity potential actually lies in fewer, not necessarily cheaper, personnel.

The reason for this is straightforward: The higher the skill level, the more flexibility the department enjoys. This concept is also known as *cross-training,* in which a flexible employee can perform a variety of tasks competently. Highly skilled and flexible employees can respond to virtually any work situation and are able to fill in for other staff. This is a very desirable quality in a fast-paced health care environment. At most organizations, it would be better to aim for a smaller but more professional and highly trained workforce than a larger, less professional, lower-wage workforce. The former option may prove to be less expensive and more satisfactory than the latter. This is not to say that high-priced professionals should do everything. It is not desirable to have RNs change bed-

ACTION	PREDICTABLE RESULT
Make the skill mix "leaner"	Cost cutting, offset by potentially • More, not fewer, employees • More supervision and training • More interruptions and handoffs • Less flexibility • Greater recruitment costs
Make the skill mix dramatically leaner	Patient care quality could suffer

Figure 1.2. Skill mix scorecard.

pans, answer every call light, and deliver every meal. There is indeed a place for the less skilled, less expensive employee, but there is a limit to how far one can push before unintended consequences push back. Figure 1.2 explains the results of the skill mix strategy.

Why is it that so many plans work out on paper but do not survive actual practice? The intersection of potentially hundreds of known and unknown variables in countless combinations could affect actual performance. Most of these variables, even when known, are often not modeled or taken into account in the financial analysis. Frequently, management has already made the decision to go ahead and orders an analysis to prove its case. Under deadline pressure, the analysis may be prepared in the simplest way possible, usually by ignoring the multitude of factors that might change the outcome and introduce a measure of uncertainty. To do otherwise might be seen as unnecessarily pessimistic and not in the best team spirit. In addition, management does not want a plan that shows ambiguous, qualified results. On the contrary, it would like to present the course of action as clear and relatively *unqualified.* People want confirmation that their instincts and judgments are correct. Ironically, in an effort to deliver certainty, the final plan may represent an improbable, best-case scenario. Certainly, it is much easier to fix a plan that has problems while still on paper than it is to fix real problems after implementation.

In an effort to check this tendency when planning, it is highly advisable to observe the following guidelines:

- *Talk to the people who will be affected.* Do they agree with the plan? Does it look achievable? If not, what are the reasons? Are these reasons legitimate, and should they be factored into the analysis? Anything that a plan might hope to achieve will have to be done through people, so get their input.

- *Perform thorough "due diligence."* Take care to evaluate the proposal from all sides: cost, quality, performance, risk factors, rates of return, human resource competencies, and so forth.

- *Do a sensitivity analysis.* Determine the major variables that could affect the outcome and what happens to the bottom-line result when any of these factors varies significantly from the expected case. Going a step further, the executives could assign a probability for each event. This would allow the organization to assess its risk and reward in a range of most probable outcomes, not just a one-point estimate.

- *Monitor the outcome.* The analysis is best structured in a way that facilitates monitoring and tracking of actual results to plan. If the plan uses factors or variables that cannot be tracked later, the factors or variables should not be used or should at least be mentioned in the narrative that accompanies the analysis so that decision makers are made aware of the risk.

- *Learn from history.* Has the organization implemented similar proposals before? What mistakes were made, and what factors contributed to success? Has this learning been thoughtfully incorporated?

What would happen if fast-paced technology companies such as Microsoft or Intel, for example, were to employ the skill mix strategy? They would replace their most experienced and skilled engineers with high-school interns and fresh graduates. They would undoubtedly have to hire more interns than the senior people they replaced. An analyst would pencil out how much that might save in salaries. The quality, however, would be terrible. No amount of interns could design, test, and manufacture the products these companies depend on. A company trying this strategy might save on salaries but arrive seriously late to market with inferior products, which would ultimately bankrupt the company. The analogy to health care is even more dramatic, as lives—not software—are at stake.

Organizations that force down the skill mix usually find that it proves to be a paper savings that never materializes, primarily because it ignores the productivity costs of segregating people and tasks. Average hourly wages per person might go down, but there may be more employees than before. This is not always the case, but organizations should avoid imposing blanket solutions for most departments where it might work only for a few. The goal, after all, is to reduce labor costs. It is a good idea to set firm labor cost standards, but there must be a great deal of flexibility granted in meeting them. Skill mix may or may not be one of them. Some managers will find that they get better overall productivity if the skill mix is a bit richer—for example, 65% of staff are RNs instead of 60%—and the economic tradeoff of higher average wages at lower total cost is worth it. Others will find that their costs are lower by matching various tasks to defined skill levels and job descriptions, making the overall skill mix leaner. Large departments, with their greater flexibility, are able to work this out much better than small ones (and therein lies a potential path to better productivity—combine small, similar departments to form larger units).

For the time being, organizations should not attempt to reengineer the skill mix. Instead, the program laid out in this book shows how to use historical analysis to develop a single cost-per-unit statistic to use as a standard. This cost standard accounts for skill mix as well as overtime and registry. That will suffice very well for now. Afterward, having achieved success with the program, some organizations may want to do something more with skill mix, but they will need a more detailed investigation of individual departments to judge the soundness of the idea. Such an exercise better fits within a benchmarking program.

BENCHMARKING

Some organizations have attempted to derive labor standards by comparing themselves with other, similar organizations. This process is commonly known as *benchmarking.* There is a lot more to benchmarking, however, than merely opening a book of comparative labor values. When comparing the productivity of one hospital with another, complex analysis is necessary to account for different patients, distinct medical practices, conflicting traditions, and unique tasks. Benchmarking is an elaborate, analytically rigorous process of discovery and adaptation—a focused approach that answers specific and fundamental questions in particular areas of the organization. Benchmarking is aimed at learning what other organizations do, how they do it, and how this knowledge can be adapted and harnessed to work at one's own organization. It is a systematic process for evaluating, comparing, and adopting industry practices recognized as best in class in order to reduce cost or enhance quality.

Quite apart from the analytical rigor that true benchmarking demands, cultural problems pose an even bigger challenge to success. In many organizations, merely adhering to department budgets proves difficult enough. Budgets attempt to encourage some discipline, yet no sooner is the budget enacted than managers begin requesting additional workers. If the discipline to adhere to an ordinary budget were lacking, how strong would the adherence to national productivity benchmarks be? Too many organizations have embarked upon this path only to be defeated by overlooked organizational problems of discipline and incentives. *Before reliable standards are firmly in place, the organization is not ready for benchmarking.*

A benchmarking company was hired to produce a report for South-western Hospital System. Southwestern's executive team was solidly behind the effort, but the department managers were vehemently opposed. They had seen what happens from such efforts when one of the big accounting firms did a "benchmarking audit" a few years before—mass layoffs. This time they would be prepared. Southwestern managers spent a lot of time "massaging" the data and disputing the veracity of the best performer peers from the benchmarking reports. When challenged by their vice-presidents to duplicate industry best performers, they instead devoted a lot of effort toward explaining how their operations and community traditions were unique, and therefore not comparable. Six months went by with no substantive productivity improvement, when the annual budget cycle again consumed everyone's time. After another round of reports one year later, Southwestern executives gave up on benchmarking and turned their attentions elsewhere.

Benchmarking is a worthwhile, highly targeted approach, one that should be attempted only after a complete productivity program has been successfully implemented. For benchmarking to be a success, managers have to be eager to do it, not have it imposed on them, which takes real teamwork and the sincere desire to improve.

Benchmarking, as usually done in the health care industry, is actually a misnomer. In reality, comparing one's own reports to a binder of reports showing "best performer" health care organizations (such as the one shown in Figure 1.3) is just a convenient starting point to identify potential benchmark partners. These reports should not simply be used to come up with labor standards to copy into the budget book. If it were indeed possible to do that, organizations could just pick the best performers, copy their labor ratios into their budgets, and be done with it. The point is that these best performer organizations and departments got that way for a good reason. They attained best performer status because there is something exceptional about their way of doing business that dis-

General Hospital A-2667
Department: **06010 MED/SURG INTENSIVE CARE**
Profile: **006010 MED/SURG ICU**
Peer Group Size: **211**
Data for Group: **<=06/30/2002**

Peer Group Criteria:
<=25000 Discharges
General Acute
Western Region
Non-Teaching
Hospital CMI <=1.500

Performance Metrics	Your Hosp A-2667	Top 5 Peer Group Performers					Performance Gap		Group Percentile Rankings			
		A-3668	A-2683	A-4670	A-8257	A-5221	Wrked Hrs	Dollars	20th	40th	60th	80th
VOLUME												
Patient Days	23,652	24,451	14,126	27,787	28,109	15,330	NA	NA	13,442	16,130	19,356	23,228
Equivalent Pt Days	24,835	25,674	14,832	29,177	29,514	16,097	NA	NA	14,114	16,937	20,324	24,389
Discharges	7,300	7,665	6,570	8,395	6,205	4,380	NA	NA	5,896	6,157	6,584	7,304
Average LOS (Days)	3.24	3.19	2.15	3.31	4.53	3.50	NA	NA	2.28	2.62	2.94	3.18
SKILL MIX												
RN	73.36%	74.09%	74.83%	80.70%	77.03%	71.89%	NA	NA	71.82%	73.72%	75.98%	78.22%
LVN	15.60%	15.76%	15.91%	14.90%	12.93%	15.29%	NA	NA	13.60%	14.22%	14.84%	15.46%
LPN	6.16%	6.22%	5.20%	0.00%	6.47%	4.20%	NA	NA	3.44%	4.06%	4.68%	5.30%
Mgmt	3.29%	3.32%	3.36%	3.62%	3.45%	3.22%	NA	NA	3.10%	3.72%	3.82%	3.92%
Other	1.59%	0.61%	0.70%	0.78%	0.12%	5.39%	NA	NA	0.58%	0.72%	0.86%	1.00%
Total	100.00%	100.00%	100.00%	100.00%	100.00%	100.00%	NA	NA	NA	NA	NA	NA
PRODUCTIVITY												
Hours Worked Per												
Patient Day	15.83	15.15	15.23	15.43	16.33	17.60	16,083	402,084	15.10	16.69	18.24	20.76
Equivalent Pt Day	15.04	14.39	14.47	14.66	15.51	16.72	15,923	398,063	14.35	15.86	17.33	19.72
Discharge	51.29	48.33	32.74	51.07	73.97	61.60	21,613	540,328	34.43	43.73	53.63	66.02
DEPARTMENT COST												
Total Cost Per												
Patient Day	474.90	454.50	456.90	462.90	489.90	528.00	NA	482,501	450.11	495.12	544.63	599.10
Equivalent Pt Day	451.16	431.78	434.06	439.76	465.41	501.60	NA	477,676	427.60	470.36	517.40	569.14
Discharge	1,538.68	1,449.86	982.34	1,532.20	2,219.25	1,848.00	NA	648,393	967.53	1,064.28	1,170.71	1,287.78

Report Date: January 2, 2003

Figure 1.3. Sample benchmarking report.

tinguishes their operating results. The job of benchmarking is to uncover those unique methods and work processes. Such knowledge, once acquired, must be adapted to the particular needs and goals of the organization, then implemented and constantly monitored for corrective action. Sound easy? The gains produced through benchmarking do not come cheaply. It would be wasteful to see those gains erode to the original situation that gave rise to the call for benchmarking in the first place.

The benchmarking process is outside the scope of this book. After completing the productivity program outlined in this book, health care organizations would do well to read up on the subject and decide if benchmarking is something that they want to attempt. Authoritative books on the subject include *The Benchmarking Book,* by Michael Spendolini, and *Business Process Benchmarking,* by Robert Camp. Neither of these books is specific to health care, but the process is the same.

PROBLEM OF OVERTIME AND REGISTRY

Overtime and registry (also called *agency*) can be a potent source of savings, yet many managers do not think they can reduce these hours. Interest in this category of "premium" labor comes and goes, depending on local labor market conditions. Nevertheless, these are expensive hours, and they add up quickly.

Many organizations have suddenly become full of patients while the number of available slots in nursing schools has remained relatively unchanged. The resulting labor shortage has produced an increasing reliance on nursing overtime and registry, the most expensive job class in the organization. It is useful to think of these categories as interchangeable because in most cases overtime and registry cost about the same, from one and one half to double "straight time" wage rates.

Premium pay, along with on-call usage and float pool "borrowing," is supposed to be incidental, filling in for occasional temporary, unforeseen gaps in scheduling, interim vacancies; unscheduled absences; sudden workload increases; and injured workers. In practice, some departments suffer high turnover in certain occupations, whereas others have inappropriate core-staffing schedules that compensate for a mismatch of staffing and workload by drawing upon overtime, on-call time, and registry. Some common reasons for staffing difficulties are

- *Inability or delay getting official approval to recruit:* Recruiting new hires can replace overtime and registry. If so, the process of filling out multiple forms, getting the necessary signoffs, and seeking approval through the official hiring committee may take weeks or even months. Delay is costly. For many managers, the path of least resistance is to authorize overtime rather than endure the new-hire process.

- *Inability to find qualified employees, inadequate recruiting effort:* Many managers privately complain that once given the official go-ahead, human resources gets bogged down in bureaucratic procedures. Conflicting priorities in human resources—managing benefits, conducting sensitivity training, equal employment opportunity instruction, payroll problems, and so forth—and possibly having budget problems of their own may explain the level of recruiting service. (Private recruitment agencies working on commission do not seem to endure the same problems.)

- *Overtime and registry hours not counted as full-time equivalents (FTEs):* At some organizations, budget procedures do not count overtime hours, registry hours, or both as labor hours and dollars. This creates a hidden incentive to use premium labor. Registry hours can be difficult to calculate when the agency submits an invoice without the number of hours worked. Even worse, registry is sometimes classified as a "purchased service," not a labor expense, and charged to a central administrative cost cen-

		Before		After			Illustration:
		Total	**Pct**	**Total**	**Pct**	**Savings**	Overtime and registry
Hours	Straight Time	2,070,000	92.0%	2,160,000	96.0%	(90,000)	reduction
	Overtime	90,000	4.0%	45,000	2.0%	45,000	made up with
	Registry	90,000	4.0%	45,000	2.0%	45,000	straight time,
	Total Hours	2,250,000	100.0%	2,250,000	100.0%	0	producing annual savings
Salaries	Straight Time	$53,076,923	87.5%	$55,384,615	93.6%	($2,307,692)	of $1.5 million
	Overtime	3,461,538	5.7%	1,730,769	2.9%	1,730,769	even though
	Registry	4,153,846	6.8%	2,076,923	3.6%	2,076,923	total hours are
	Total Salaries	$60,692,308	100.0%	$59,192,308	100.0%	$1,500,000	unchanged
Hourly Wages	Straight Time	$25.64	95.1%	$25.64	97.5%	$0.00	
	Overtime	38.46	4.0%	38.46	2.0%	0.00	
	Registry	46.15	4.0%	46.15	2.0%	0.00	
	Average Wage	$26.97	100.0%	$26.31	100.0%	$0.67	

Figure 1.4. Sample overtime and registry analysis.

ter. Managers' true productivity performance can thus escape the otherwise vigilant eyes of the budget police.

• *Reluctance of managers to hire for fear of low census days:* Low census days (i.e., days with few patients) are (or should be) a relatively rare occurrence. It is not sensible to keep the core staffing schedule low and then staff with overtime in order to avoid the small chance of a low census day. It may not be the kindest act to send employees home on slower days, but that is part of the manager's job. If low census days are frequent, departments ought to be combined to bring up the census and enable more efficient staffing levels.

Sample Overtime and Registry Analysis

The continual use of premium labor represents a serious cost control problem. As a rule, if premium labor is used regularly to the extent of one FTE or more for any given department, it is cheaper to hire a permanent, straight-time replacement. This would have no impact

Suzanne is the department manager for a busy intermediate care nursing department. The busy season is upon her, and some of her experienced staff members have been getting better offers elsewhere, including substantial signing bonuses. She wants to match these offers, but the answer has been no, and she will soon have vacancies in a tight labor market. The alternative is to call the agency, but she figures it will actually end up costing more than meeting the market. Overtime is a possibility to plug the gap, but the cost is almost as prohibitive. Her hospital now pays incentives to recruit new nurses, but not to retain existing staff. Still, that is an administrative decision, not her own. She only hopes that administration will not give her trouble about exceeding the budget.

on productivity, measured as hours per unit of service, but a big impact on cost. Figure 1.4 is a quick analysis that gives the organization an estimate of the potential savings opportunity. In this analysis, there is no change in productivity, as the number of FTEs before and after is the same. Only the cost is different.

To keep the exercise realistic, select for the analysis only those departments that have relied on overtime and registry to the degree of at least one FTE on a regular basis over an extended time, say 6–12 months. It is safe to assume that departments using less than an FTE's worth of labor have overtime and registry under control. The analysis answers the question of how much money the organization could save by replacing its premium staff with the same number of regular staff at straight-time pay. This analysis covers the whole facility or health care system, and uses average straight time, overtime and registry wage rates. After this quick analysis, the same analysis would be done for each department, using department-specific hourly wages.

In Figure 1.4, overtime and registry are reduced in half, from a combined 8% of total hours to 4% of total hours. Increasing straight time hours so that total hours are the same in each case makes up the difference. The illustration shows annual savings of $1.5 million, even though total hours are unchanged.

This is a conservative estimate of the savings potential because in-house replacement staff might not always be exchanged one-for-one with overtime and registry staff. Cross-training, job-sharing, and other strategies explored below could reduce the demand for overtime and registry labor, and the organization could do much better than a simple one-for-one replacement.

There are additional important benefits to weigh. Registry personnel impose a hidden burden on training and orientation time, which costs money. While training, registry personnel simply cannot be as productive as regular, experienced employees can. They cannot know the organization as well, nor can they perform to expectations in a short time. Once they are trained and performing satisfactorily, they might leave for another assignment, and the process starts over with new people. Of course, large, hidden training costs are not unique to registry personnel. Turnover of regular employees also keeps the organization paying constantly for training new recruits, as well as keeping the demand high for overtime and registry to fill in during recruiting.

Aside from the cost, having employees work overtime on a regular basis is problematic. Most workers in high-stress areas cannot function as effectively in the overtime hours as they do on the opening hours of their shift. Tired employees are not as productive. To the extent possible, departments should identify where overtime hours can be replaced with new hires. It is less expensive and more useful to the department.

Strategies for Reducing Overtime and Registry

Departments with low turnover and few unscheduled absences have reduced need for overtime, registry, or recruitment of new employees. Such departments demonstrate good morale, good pay practices, or both. Conversely, departments with high turnover and frequent unscheduled absences have more need of overtime and spend resources recruiting new employees. Departments like these may experience poor morale or have substandard pay practices. Another possibility is inappropriate core-staffing schedules that compensate for a mismatch of staffing and workload by drawing upon overtime, on-call time, and registry to close the gap.

A successful strategy for reducing the reliance on overtime and registry should aim to realize these goals:

1. *Low turnover:* Employees leaving to work elsewhere (usually the competition!) should serve as a warning sign to managers that there are unresolved problems with working conditions. Happy employees do not leave for greener pastures. The core reasons for these troubles should be surveyed and then corrected, not ignored.

2. *Few unscheduled absences:* Although employees are entitled to occasional sick days, they are not entitled to an excessive number of unscheduled absences. Frequent unscheduled absences point to morale problems or problem employees. The former is a management issue, the latter a disciplinary issue.

3. *Few workplace injuries:* The personal and monetary costs of injuries are high. It may pay the organization to consult with an expert to redesign tasks to be less hazardous and physically strenuous.

4. *Good pay practices:* People have to be paid at market rate, even when a market for some classes of employees exists outside the health care industry, such as kitchen workers, computer technicians, engineers, accountants, secretaries, and many others. If not, an incentive to quit is created, and the best, most marketable employees are the first to go.

5. *Appropriate core-staffing schedules:* In patient care departments, a core-staffing schedule geared to actual workloads may not have been addressed for a while, although patient volume may have

grown considerably. The gap between the core-staffing schedule and reality may have been filled with premium labor.

Even in tight labor markets, it is a mistake to assume that nothing can be done to reduce premium labor. Excessive overtime and registry are symptoms of breakdowns somewhere in the above areas, and fixing these problems will go a long way toward reducing the demand for overtime and registry.

Float Pools

Float pools are comprised of employees who have the training and experience to *float* to whatever department can use them. These pools are often used not only as replacements for temporary vacancies and absences but also as a training ground for permanent positions. The float pool acts as a kind of relief valve that allows departments to avoid much overtime. Float pool employees are also sometimes used to cover for staffing and morale problems in various departments. When floats are utilized not as back-up for temporary conditions, but as steady employees, one or more of the five problems listed previously is most likely present.

If float pool employees are not offered full benefits like other staffers, they can be hard to recruit, but that is easy to change. The goal should not be to save money on benefits but to replace chronic overtime and registry with regular, long-term (straight-time) employees. Anything that will further this end should be encouraged to ensure adequate, steady pools.

Another possibility to promote a flexible, highly trained staffing pool is to elevate the float pool to an elite, professional career track. Multi-skilled individuals who can work anywhere represent a considerable asset to the organization, and it is worth paying more to get this kind of employee. Float pools should not be considered merely as a temporary training ground when their potential is for so much more.

HOSPITAL MERGERS

Many mergers are motivated by the desire to eliminate excess capacity and form a more efficient organization. In pursuit of efficiency, many hospitals that merge into health care systems often look for excess administration as a place to cut costs. Because clinical staff will still be needed to care for patients, eliminating unnecessary administrative duplication is often anticipated as the key area in which the combined entity might cut costs. Proposed "economies of scale" may be cited. This might seem like a good idea, but such an approach is not destined to yield much fruit for four often-overlooked reasons:

1. *The majority of labor costs are clinical, not administrative.* Unless there is radical overhaul of administrative functions—which the organization could do without a merger—there is probably not enough savings to be realized at the administrative level alone to change unfavorable hospital economics. With some exceptions, middle and senior management costs are a small part of total costs. Today, most middle managers are also "working" managers anyway, doing staff work and quality control most of the time. Whatever costs can be saved are seldom sufficient or enduring enough on their own to justify the trouble and upheaval of merging into a health care system.

Performance Measure	Hospitals by Bed Size, 2000					
	100–199	200–299	300–399	400–499	>499	All Hospitals
Inpatient Hours per Discharge[1]	115.0	114.6	121.9	111.3	113.4	116.3
Outpatient Hours per Visit	6.4	6.1	6.2	7.5	6.5	6.2
Compensation Costs per Discharge[2]	2,622	2,634	2,866	2,609	2,708	2,638

[1]Case mix adjusted
[2]Wage index and Case mix adjusted

Median values from Almanac of Hospital & Financial Operating Indicators ©2002 Ingenix, Inc.

Figure 1.5.   Performance of large hospitals versus small hospitals.

2. *Mergers impose new layers of cost.* The new, larger institution will almost certainly impose certain costs of its own—new levels of reporting and management, integration of information, reporting, billing, financial systems, and so forth. A "corporate tax" or levy on the system's hospitals usually funds these "corporate services."

3. *Bigger is not always better.* It might seem reasonable to consolidate many overhead administrative functions, such as billing, financial planning, marketing, and so forth. Much is made of so-called "economies of scale," the idea that as a business grows, it gets more efficient. Is that true? Look at the evidence: Except for hospitals smaller than 100 beds (not shown), Figure 1.5 does not demonstrate any superiority for large hospitals compared with small hospitals. One of the reasons undoubtedly stems from the scheduling, communication, and coordination problems that come with size. Past a certain point, economies of scale work in reverse. Bigger is not necessarily better, and it may even cost more.

4. *Customer service levels decrease with size.* The bigger the unit, the worse the service, and this tends to be especially true when administrative functions are centralized for various hospitals within corporate headquarters. As a business grows, its size works against customer intimacy. When services are centralized at corporate headquarters, intimate customer contact is easily lost. With many hospitals to serve, corporate administrators concern themselves with standardization, making it easier for them to keep control and compare operating results. Corporate administrators begin to prescribe what services will be offered and at what price (the corporate tax). What an individual hospital wants becomes secondary. Over time, it becomes increasingly likely that services the hospital provides for itself, at its own cost, will better meet its individual needs than what it

may get with a centralized corporate office serving numerous other hospitals.

Market-Based Solution

Health care system executives may seldom hear any complaints from their client hospitals that the corporate tax is an undue burden. It is not politically astute for a hospital to do a feasibility study of providing a centralized corporate service for itself, tailored precisely to its own specifications, at a cost it deems reasonable. Even less politically astute would be a hospital proposing not to purchase the corporate service at all, saving the money for other purposes.

Facilities with a system pay the cost of centralized services as a corporate "tax," a monthly charge for corporate overhead. The tax is frequently levied without regard to actual use, as would be the case if use were charged on a time and materials basis or from a fee schedule. Corporate services are a sunk cost, an automatic expense regardless of use. It is, therefore, in each hospital's interest to secure more centralized services of particular benefit to itself because other hospitals share in the cost, even if they receive no benefit. The reverse is also true: It is not in any hospital's self-interest to reduce its own demand for corporate services, even if it were offered the option. The savings would be trivial, as they, too, would presumably be shared. This situation generates the classic cost spiral, fueled when customers demand unlimited quantities of free goods. At the other end, the corporate office interprets the strong demand for its centralized services as a signal to expand! With expansion, the cost of these services swells and boosts the corporate tax on each client facility, threatening the profitability of the whole system.

This is a classic problem of knowledge and incentives. The corporate office has no knowledge of its customers' true demand for its services so long as the customers are compelled to pay regardless of whether they want services or use a lot or a little. Because the client facilities have to pay, they have no incentive to reduce demand for more corporate-provided services. The corporate office interprets this demand for more "free" corporate services as strong approval of central planning. Logically, there is no other way for them to interpret this situation. There is no way to know exactly what services are desired, and no way to discern a fair, market price (as opposed to passing through costs) if there are no real, paying customers.

Why not position corporate services as a real business by offering real customers the services they freely desire and billing directly by invoice? Offer facilities the option of purchasing corporate services and paying directly for them, or withdrawing and providing the services themselves, through other parties, or not at all, as appropriate. True value at competitive prices would emerge. Such a move would revolutionize the relationship between headquarters and client facilities. If not enough client facilities were to buy the corporate offering to make it feasible, then the service would either be dropped or revamped to make it more attractive, just like a real business. If the corporate service were well subscribed, this would indicate satisfied customers paying for services they desire at mutually agreeable prices. If cost reduction and service are important, health care systems should look into a market-based solution.

> "THE GREAT THING IN THIS WORLD IS NOT SO MUCH WHERE WE ARE BUT IN WHAT DIRECTION WE ARE MOVING."
> —OLIVER WENDELL HOLMES

SUMMARY

Despite the focus on productivity, most "solutions" devised prove to be fleeting. Every organization seems to have its own approach to managing productivity. Under the surface, however, this is not the case. There are fundamental problems that must be solved before productivity can really be managed. These include excessive reliance on budgets, overly complex measurement systems that confound understanding, no clear accountability, lack of authority at the right management level, short review cycles that emphasize statistical variation, no incentives to improve, and no disincentives to prevent decline.

Layoffs do not work. Although staff can always be eliminated, it is much more difficult to do away with their work. Backlogs begin accumulating, the quality of care may deteriorate, and employee morale is hurt. The predictable result: staffing slowly increases to former levels. The initial savings quickly disappear. The preferred course emphasizes planning and continually adjusting labor resources to work demands so that a layoff is unnecessary.

Skill mix refers to the average level of training, certification, and experience in departments. The organization's skill mix can be made leaner, but this should be approached with caution. Skill mix changes look attractive on paper, but unintended consequences of supervision, workflow, efficiency, and clinical outcomes often surface. At most organizations, it would be better to aim for a smaller, more professional, highly trained workforce than a larger, less professional, lower-wage workforce. The former option may prove to be less expensive and more satisfactory.

Benchmarking is an analytically rigorous process to solve problems of service, cost, or cycle times. The job of benchmarking is to uncover unique methods and work processes that yield superior operating results. Such knowledge must be adapted to the particular needs and goals of the organization, implemented, and constantly monitored for corrective action. This process should not be confused with a binder of reports showing best performer organizations. Such reports are just a convenient starting point to identify potential benchmark partners. Before organizations have tackled basic productivity problems, they are not ready for benchmarking.

Overtime and registry are more expensive than many organizations may realize. A simple analysis can assess the cost reduction potential. Contributing factors include inability to or delay in getting official approval to recruit; inability to find qualified employees and/or inadequate recruiting effort; and overtime and registry hours not officially counted as FTEs. Strategies for reducing overtime and registry must address both the demand side and the supply side of the equation. These include lowering staff turnover, minimizing unscheduled absences, instituting good pay practices, and developing appropriate core-staffing schedules.

Centralizing administrative functions can result in extra labor cost and worse service, the opposite of what is intended. This is mainly due to four reasons: the majority of labor costs are clinical rather than administrative, mergers impose new layers of cost, bigger is not always better, and customer service levels tend to decrease with size. A market-based solution is offered as an alternative to mandated corporate overhead.

HOW TO
DEVELOP REALISTIC
PRODUCTIVITY
STANDARDS

A *labor standard* is a productivity measure that relates workload to staffing. Realistic labor standards, acceptable to department managers, form the foundation of superior productivity. This chapter demonstrates how to develop practical standards by mining the organization's history.

Learn from History

Some organizations have attempted to derive labor standards by comparing themselves with other organizations. As mentioned in

Chapter 1, this process is commonly known as benchmarking, but there is a lot more to benchmarking than a book of comparative labor values. When comparing the productivity of one organization with another, complex analysis is necessary to account for different patients, distinct medical practices, and unique tasks. Too many organizations have embarked on this path only to be defeated by overlooked organizational problems of discipline and incentives.

A much more effective alternative, one that avoids such an analytical problem, is to mine the organization's own history. By comparing each department's performance over several years to its current performance, most of the concerns that prevent real improvement are eliminated. Using historical analysis, many organizations will find that productivity has slipped over time, and this can be reversed. History serves as a very accurate guide to the organization's potential for productivity improvement.

Because the focus is on current performance compared to history, the analysis ignores whether departments met their productivity targets. Whether they achieved a 100% score against some standard of budgeted performance is of no consequence. Budgets are different from year to year, and it is therefore possible for a department to hit its targets every year and yet to have a *worse* actual record of performance than the year before.

Assign Performance Measures

To start, workload measures, or "units of service," should be assigned for every department, including the traditionally "fixed" departments, whose staffing is set without regard to readily measurable work volume. The unit of service describes a department's mission, its purpose, or its patients. Examples include patient days, visits, procedures, treatments, and cases. Usually these measures will be long established and convenient to use. It is generally preferable to use the workload units already in use because these measures have a history and familiarity in the departments and throughout the organization. Relating the growth of fixed departments to that of the overall organization is a useful indirect measure (hospital volume is commonly expressed as *adjusted discharges* or *adjusted patient days*).

Some managers may be concerned that their unit of service does not capture all of the various tasks that department staff members perform, such as charting, filling out logs, reporting, answering call lights, talking to patients' families, and so forth. If the unit of service is carefully selected, however, this is not true. The unit of service is a measure of a department's main *output* or *service*, not its *inputs or tasks*. If the unit of service is patient days, for example, then all of the tasks associated with the care of patients make up the unit of service, from admission work up to discharge planning and everything in between. The output measure of patient days captures all the related activities. If the unit of service is tests, but personnel also prepare reports, attend meetings, and make follow-up calls, then the number of tests will capture all the associated tasks. This is the final output, and it is what the customer is paying for. If everything associated with taking care of the patient is included in hours worked, then all of the tasks are being counted. It is not necessary or even desirable to count every activity individually, not only because of the extra burden of record-keeping but also to avoid introducing an unintended incentive to perform more activities, when the goal ought to be simplifying and reducing the number of activities required for patient care.

Whatever the measure, department managers must agree that their unit of service is appropriate. If they do not, then other measures should be substituted until agreement is reached. Even though finding new measures may prove somewhat inconvenient and time consuming, it will greatly aid acceptance. Without acceptance, compliance to the goals of the productivity program will suffer. The ultimate outcome is 100% compliance throughout the entire organization. That is an entirely realistic goal if the program is designed and executed with reason and logic. Anything that can be done to ensure success is worth whatever price must be paid in speed.

Performance Measures for the Entire Organization

Although each department has its own performance measure, what measure is best to use for the whole organization? How does an organization measure its overall performance? There are three main measures in use by hospitals today.

1. Labor hours per adjusted discharge
2. Labor hours per adjusted patient day
3. Full-time equivalent (FTE) employees per adjusted occupied bed (another way of expressing labor hours per adjusted patient day, except that hours are converted to FTE, and adjusted patients days are divided by 365 to get adjusted occupied beds)

The workload indicator of the entire hospital is patients, but there are inpatients and outpatients, and equating the two is problematic. Inpatients consume vastly different amounts of resources than outpatients; how are the two equated for a single measure of hospital workload? The "adjustment" on each of the three measures is an approximation that equates outpatients to inpatients by using the relative amounts of gross charges for each (also called *gross revenue*). The formula is

Discharges (or patient days), times total gross hospital charges, divided by inpatient gross charges

The ratio of total gross charges to inpatient gross charges yields a multiplier that is applied to inpatient discharges or inpatient days. This multiplier is the adjustment factor. It is immediately obvious that the multiplier is a major determinant of the final number of adjusted discharges or days. Furthermore, how the hospital sets its outpatient prices relative to its inpatient prices affects the multiplier. If a health care organization were to raise its outpatient prices while leaving its inpatient prices alone, the multiplier would rise, and there would be more adjusted discharges or adjusted patient days from the price change alone. Suppose, for example, that a health care organization raises its outpatient prices 10%, with no

		Before	After	Change
Pricing Structure	Outpatient Charges	50	55	10.0%
Dollars in Millions	Inpatient Charges	100	100	0.0%
	Total Hospital Charges	**150**	**155**	**3.3%**
	Total Charges to Inpatient Charges	1.50	1.55	3.3%
Effect on Patient Volume	Inpatient Discharges	20,000	20,000	0.0%
	x Adjustment Factor	1.50	1.55	3.3%
	Adjusted Discharges	**30,000**	**31,000**	**3.3%**
	Patient Days	80,000	80,000	0.0%
	x Adjustment Factor	1.50	1.55	3.3%
	Adjusted Patient Days	**120,000**	**124,000**	**3.3%**

Figure 2.1. Pricing structure and its effect on patient volume.

change in inpatient prices, as illustrated in Figure 2.1. The actual numbers of patients are the same.

In this example, raising outpatient prices by 10% has the effect of boosting adjusted discharges and adjusted patient days 3.3%, even though the actual numbers of patients are the same before as after. A 3.3% increase in adjusted discharges is a large increase. When organizations were mainly inpatient oriented, the adjustment factor was not as critical. If an organization earned only 10% of its gross revenue from outpatients, any change in the adjustment factor from year to year was relatively small and any distortion in the number of adjusted discharges minimal. Today, when one third or more of gross revenues might be outpatient, the effect of any relative change in prices is magnified.

As long as the hospital increases its inpatient and outpatient prices by the same percentage (i.e., the adjustment multiplier is the same), the ratio is not especially troublesome. As long as the pricing structure is consistent, the comparison of one year to the next is valid, whether by overall adjusted discharges or adjusted patient days. There is no reason, however, to think that a health care organization is, or even should be, consistent in its pricing structure. The goal of gross price adjustments is to increase net revenue, not to keep the adjustment factor constant. Simply using the same adjustment multiplier would not work either because, unlike the hypothetical example, the real number of inpatients and outpatients do change every year and must be accounted for.

The point of this exercise is to demonstrate that adjusted discharges and adjusted patient days may not be a good workload indicator to use in a productivity calculation. Until someone comes up with something better, however, it is all that hospitals have available to measure their overall progress in improving their productivity. Organizations should keep in mind two points:

- Adjusted discharges and adjusted patient days should be interpreted for reasonable consistency from year to year before using them to calculate total organization productivity.

- Productivity is improved department by department, not at the total organization level. The best way to measure the effect of improving productivity is to sum each department's results. Adjusted discharges and adjusted days are useful only as a shorthand measure.

Do the Math

Combining workload with hours and salaries determines each department's productivity loss or gain for several years. Hours and salaries are then divided by workload to yield productivity ratios. These ratios are then applied to *current* workload volumes and compared with *current* productivity levels. The results reveal the savings each department could achieve by operating at a better standard of performance—a standard that had once been achieved and is therefore repeatable (with some exceptions, as discussed later in this chapter).

Each department's productivity should be compared to itself over several years. Current *actual* performance is compared to historical *actual* performance on a completely variable basis for every department, no matter whether the department is classified as *fixed* or *variable*. The objective is not to compare how departments did against their budgets, but how they performed over time.

How to Prepare the Analysis

For each department, the analyst gathers the following statistics:

- Annual and year-to-date units of service (if unavailable or not applicable, adjusted discharges should be used to compare the growth of the department against the growth of the organization)
- Annual and year-to-date productive (or "worked") hours and wages, including overtime, registry, and temporary hours and dollars

Annualized year-to-date figures must be based on at least 3 months of history. Any less, and the reliability compared to prior years is compromised. Once these statistics are at hand, the analyst would arrange them in the format depicted in Figure 2.2.

Illustration: 3-Year Productivity Analysis

A nursing unit analysis appears in Figure 2.2. Hours per patient day were 12.0 in 2000, and then improved (i.e., declined) to 11.9 hours per patient day in 2001. The productivity improvement saved the organization 512 hours. In 2002, productivity dived to 12.8 hours per patient day, costing the organization an additional 2,910 hours. To quantify the financial impact of the productivity lost since 2001, the increase in hours worked per patient day in 2002 (0.9) is multiplied by 2002 (current) workload volume. In this nursing unit example, the analysis reveals a productivity improvement of $15,653 in 2001 over the prior year, but a $93,348 loss in 2002. The appropriate goal is to reverse the productivity loss that occurred in 2002, accomplished by returning the department to its performance of 11.9 hours worked per patient day achieved in 2001.

When 20 or 30 departments are in this same situation, as is often the case, there are serious savings to pursue. How can this be done? The rest of this book explores the policies and procedures needed to turn potential savings into reality.

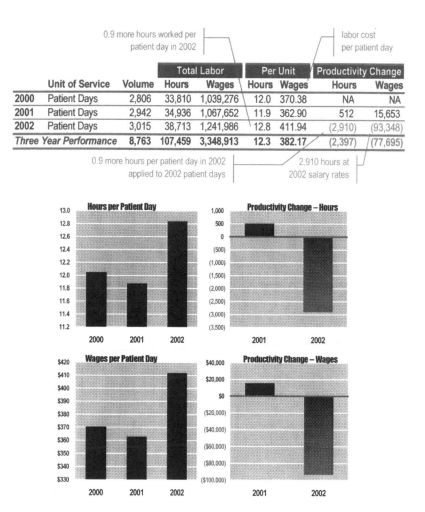

Figure 2.2. Three-year department productivity analysis.

The analysis uses "productive" or worked hours and wages only, excluding vacation, sick, and holiday. Employees are entitled to varying amounts of vacation, and sick time is unpredictable, so there is no point in including these employee benefits in the department analysis. It is best to estimate their effect at the total organization level. Vacation, sick leave, holiday pay, and employee benefits such as health insurance and payroll taxes add about one third to productive wages. If the analysis showed that $3 million in productive wage savings could be realized for the entire organization, for example, then adding one third to this sum would mean $4 million in savings when employee benefits are included.

For each department, it is essential to include those hours and dollars spent on registry and temporary employees. Not doing so excludes a significant fraction of many departments' workforces, throwing off the analysis, making departments look more productive than they really were. Another issue is the restructuring of cost centers during the period of the analysis, in which people and func-

---

How to do the Calculations:

Productive Hours per Unit of Service: productive hours divided by workload volume.

Productive Wages per Unit of Service: productive dollars divided by workload volume.

Productivity Change: Productive Hours: current year productive hours per unit of service, minus last year's productive hours per unit of service, multiplied by current year workload volume.

Productivity Change—Productive Wages: multiply the productive hours in the column to the left by average hourly wages (including temporary worker and registry). Total productive dollars divided by total productive hours, equals average hourly wages.

---

tions formerly assigned to one cost center are split amongst several. The best way to deal with this is to recombine cost centers for the analysis and make them whole. Suppose Medical Records and Coding were combined, for example, but then later split into two distinct cost centers. Without adjusting for this fact, the productivity of each cost center would look remarkably improved from prior years. Combined for the analysis, the problem goes away.

Don't Forget Registry

Many organizations do not track registry hours, just the dollar amount of the invoices. Even worse, some organizations place all registry expenses into a centralized administrative department where they entirely disappear from department cost center reports. This practice raises an automatic red flag. Given that registry employees are among the most expensive in the organization, this relaxed accounting approach simply will not do. It is impossible to know the true state of productivity in a department when a meaningful portion of its labor resources is absent. In addition, swings in registry usage from year to year will throw off the productivity comparisons if registry is omitted.

This situation often arises as an unintended consequence of the budgeting system in use. In an effort to control labor costs, attention is directed to payroll employees. If registry hours are not reported, it is very convenient for department managers to meet their budget allocation by calling the agency. The accounting department, if it is at all inclined to gather such data, must calculate and log agency hours as a manual entry. Given that no one may ask for it, least of all the department manager, it is easy for registry labor to escape notice.

The logical approach is to ignore the source of the labor. Aside from some qualitative problems that may arise from excessive reliance on agencies, the only difference between a health care organization employee drawing a salary from payroll and a registry employee drawing a paycheck from the agency is simply one of relative cost. Labor from any source must be counted as hours worked in each department in order to match hours with workload.

If this is not already the practice, a sensible approach involves collecting the hours worked for each agency by year, then calculating an average hourly rate by dividing one into the other. The average hourly rate is then divided into the monthly invoice to get the number of agency hours. If this proves too onerous, a sampling of agency invoices and hours billed can be used to calculate a reasonably accurate rate. If the agencies cannot be persuaded to include the number of hours billed on each invoice, this calculated rate can be used each month as the agency bills arrive to derive registry hours. The accountants who log these invoices can easily be trained to book the appropriate hours as well.

Float Pool

Float pool labor should be accurately coded to the departments in which each "floater" has worked. Floaters should code 100% of their time to the departments where they worked, so that each month the balance in the float pool cost center is zero or very close. If a balance were to remain, it would mean that managers spread the true cost of their own department's labor around. It follows that there should be no hours or dollars budgeted for the float pool.

Communicating the Findings

Arranging the departments' analyses in descending order of productivity lost serves to focus senior management attention where it is most needed. The first pages are the most important, allowing the reader to get to the point quickly and keep the highest priorities in plain view.

Grouping each department into one of four sections can increase emphasis still more:

1. *Losing ground*—departments whose productivity has worsened

2. *Holding steady*—departments whose productivity is roughly the same over the study period

3. *Gaining*—departments whose productivity has improved

4. *New programs and other*—new departments or services, grant-funded services, clinical research programs, and so forth

Three Year Labor Performance

			Total Labor		Per Unit		Productivity Change	
	Unit of Service	Volume	Hours	Wages	Hours	Wages	Hours	Wages
ER+Urgent Care								
2000	Visit Equiv	36,667	75,596	1,883,879	2.1	51.38	0	0
2001	Visit Equiv	43,656	105,104	2,471,231	2.4	56.61	(15,099)	(355,008)
2002	Visit Equiv	47,853	130,707	3,119,417	2.7	65.19	(15,499)	(369,887)
Three Year Performance		128,176	311,407	7,474,527	2.4	58.31	(30,598)	(724,895)
West Three								
2000	Equiv Pt Days	10,437	100,257	2,114,789	9.6	202.62	0	0
2001	Equiv Pt Days	11,095	114,730	2,321,297	10.3	209.22	(8,151)	(164,927)
2002	Equiv Pt Days	11,007	115,684	2,504,220	10.5	227.51	(1,864)	(40,358)
Three Year Performance		32,539	330,671	6,940,306	10.2	213.29	(10,016)	(205,285)
Pharmacy								
2000	1000 Billed Doses	61,990	51,369	1,121,047	0.8	18.08	0	0
2001	1000 Billed Doses	72,029	58,187	1,227,369	0.8	17.04	1,502	31,675
2002	1000 Billed Doses	76,333	71,576	1,608,028	0.9	21.07	(9,912)	(222,690)
Three Year Performance		210,352	181,132	3,956,444	0.9	18.81	(8,411)	(191,015)
Labor+Delivery								
2000	RVUs	9,935	62,871	1,478,088	6.3	148.78	0	0
2001	RVUs	10,734	68,716	1,625,570	6.4	151.44	(789)	(18,654)
2002	RVUs	11,232	76,261	1,805,115	6.8	160.71	(4,358)	(103,144)
Three Year Performance		31,901	207,848	4,908,773	6.5	153.88	(5,146)	(121,798)

(continued)

Three Year Labor Performance

		Unit of Service	Volume	Total Labor		Per Unit		Productivity Change	
				Hours	Wages	Hours	Wages	Hours	Wages
Engineering	2000	100 Gross Feet	5,124	33,306	631,341	6.5	123.21	0	0
	2001	100 Gross Feet	5,124	33,767	663,692	6.6	129.53	(461)	(9,064)
	2002	100 Gross Feet	5,124	36,175	730,701	7.1	142.60	(2,408)	(48,644)
	Three Year Performance		15,372	103,249	2,025,734	6.7	131.78	(2,869)	(57,708)
Surgery	2000	100 Surg Min	6,708	73,415	1,626,691	10.9	242.50	0	0
	2001	100 Surg Min	7,166	75,052	1,672,639	10.5	233.41	3,376	75,228
	2002	100 Surg Min	7,212	80,377	1,895,847	11.1	262.87	(4,843)	(114,237)
	Three Year Performance		21,086	228,844	5,195,177	10.9	246.38	(1,468)	(39,008)
Imaging	2000	Procedures	60,880	30,440	341,218	0.5	5.60	0	0
	2001	Procedures	67,613	34,483	425,457	0.5	6.29	(676)	(8,342)
	2002	Procedures	66,686	35,215	460,049	0.5	6.90	(1,205)	(15,744)
	Three Year Performance		195,179	100,138	1,226,724	0.5	6.29	(1,881)	(24,086)
Total	2000			427,255	9,197,053	NA	NA	0	0
	2001			490,038	10,407,255	NA	NA	(20,299)	(449,092)
	2002			545,996	12,123,377	NA	NA	(40,090)	(914,705)
	Three Year Performance			1,463,289	31,727,685	NA	NA	(60,389)	(1,363,797)

Figure 2.3. Performance of the losing ground group.

Three Year Labor Performance

		Unit of Service	Volume	Total Labor		Per Unit		Productivity Change	
				Hours	Wages	Hours	Wages	Hours	Wages
O/P Surgery	2000	100 OR Minutes	2,451	27,615	581,958	11.3	237.44	0	0
	2001	100 OR Minutes	2,862	30,835	640,497	10.8	223.79	1,411	29,302
	2002	100 OR Minutes	2,830	31,742	705,842	11.2	249.41	(1,252)	(27,835)
	Three Year Performance		8,143	90,192	1,928,297	11.1	236.80	159	1,467
Outreach	2000	Adj Discharges	16,808	10,216	124,515	0.6	7.41	0	0
	2001	Adj Discharges	18,840	11,224	135,842	0.6	7.21	227	2,748
	2002	Adj Discharges	20,441	12,305	158,038	0.6	7.73	(127)	(1,634)
	Three Year Performance		56,089	33,745	418,395	0.6	7.46	100	1,114
Print & Mail	2000	100 Copies	37,949	2,001	21,980	0.1	0.58	0	0
	2001	100 Copies	39,399	2,022	22,721	0.1	0.58	55	623
	2002	100 Copies	37,949	2,092	24,362	0.1	0.64	(144)	(1,682)
	Three Year Performance		115,297	6,115	69,063	0.1	0.60	(89)	(1,059)

(continued)

Three Year Labor Performance

		Volume	Total Labor		Per Unit		Productivity Change	
	Unit of Service		Hours	Wages	Hours	Wages	Hours	Wages
Nutrition								
2000	Consults	11,028	16,873	255,524	1.5	23.17	0	0
2001	Consults	12,259	17,408	270,898	1.4	22.10	1,348	20,985
2002	Consults	12,300	18,942	284,308	1.5	23.11	(1,476)	(22,154)
Three Year Performance		**35,587**	**53,223**	**810,730**	**1.5**	**22.78**	**(128)**	**(1,169)**
Radiology								
2000	Procedures	30,586	22,634	412,924	0.7	13.50	0	0
2001	Procedures	34,071	24,190	448,189	0.7	13.15	1,022	18,938
2002	Procedures	33,548	24,826	472,621	0.7	14.09	(1,006)	(19,160)
Three Year Performance		**98,205**	**71,650**	**1,333,734**	**0.7**	**13.58**	**16**	**(223)**
Total								
2000			79,338	1,396,901	NA	NA	0	0
2001			85,679	1,518,147	NA	NA	4,064	72,596
2002			89,907	1,645,171	NA	NA	(4,006)	(72,465)
Three Year Performance			**254,924**	**4,560,219**	**NA**	**NA**	**58**	**131**

Figure 2.4. Performance of the holding steady group.

Three Year Labor Performance

		Unit of Service	Volume	Total Labor		Per Unit		Productivity Change	
				Hours	Wages	Hours	Wages	Hours	Wages
Gaining									
Kitchen	2000	100 Meals Served	5,182	97,681	1,151,026	18.9	222.12	0	0
	2001	100 Meals Served	6,670	97,515	1,173,470	14.6	175.93	28,214	339,520
	2002	100 Meals Served	6,575	96,127	1,198,372	14.6	182.26	0	0
	Three Year Performance		18,427	291,323	3,522,868	15.8	191.18	28,214	339,520
Housekeeping	2000	100 Ft Cleaned	3,258	92,428	1,009,241	28.4	309.77	0	0
	2001	100 Ft Cleaned	3,054	67,034	763,865	21.9	250.12	19,607	223,421
	2002	100 Ft Cleaned	3,224	72,287	862,098	22.4	267.40	(1,522)	(18,146)
	Three Year Performance		9,536	231,749	2,635,204	24.3	276.34	18,085	205,275
Purchasing	2000	Adj Discharges	16,808	65,493	839,963	3.9	49.97	0	0
	2001	Adj Discharges	18,840	64,318	855,273	3.4	45.40	8,969	119,267
	2002	Adj Discharges	20,441	67,455	938,262	3.3	45.90	2,329	32,393
	Three Year Performance		56,089	197,267	2,633,498	3.5	46.95	11,298	151,660
Coronary Care	2000	Patient Days	2,162	57,123	1,526,033	26.4	705.84	0	0
	2001	Patient Days	2,129	58,365	1,559,789	27.4	732.64	(2,114)	(56,493)
	2002	Patient Days	2,367	57,199	1,545,496	24.2	652.93	7,691	207,815
	Three Year Performance		6,658	172,688	4,631,318	25.9	695.60	5,577	151,322

(continued)

Three Year Labor Performance

		Unit of Service	Volume	Total Labor		Per Unit		Productivity Change	
				Hours	Wages	Hours	Wages	Hours	Wages
Business Office	2000	100 Orig Claims	947	43,410	550,268	45.8	531.06	0	0
	2001	100 Orig Claims	1,220	44,628	592,993	36.6	436.06	11,297	150,112
	2002	100 Orig Claims	1,275	50,477	703,211	39.6	551.54	(3,838)	(53,465)
	Three Year Performance		3,442	138,515	1,846,472	40.2	536.45	7,459	96,648
Laboratory	2000	100 Billed Tests	2,259	70,303	1,278,568	31.1	566.07	0	0
	2001	100 Billed Tests	2,387	69,782	1,299,088	29.2	544.29	4,508	83,925
	2002	100 Billed Tests	2,623	76,825	1,405,277	29.3	535.81	(145)	(2,646)
	Three Year Performance		7,268	216,909	3,982,933	29.8	548.00	4,363	81,279
Admitting 8561	2000	100 Registrations	971	46,288	571,962	47.7	589.04	0	0
	2001	100 Registrations	1,170	45,911	587,994	39.2	502.56	9,863	126,320
	2002	100 Registrations	1,200	51,300	664,646	42.8	553.87	(4,212)	(54,571)
	Three Year Performance		3,341	143,498	1,824,602	43.0	546.12	5,651	71,749
Total	2000			472,726	6,927,061	NA	NA	0	0
	2001			447,553	6,832,472	NA	NA	80,344	986,071
	2002			471,670	7,317,362	NA	NA	304	111,381
	Three Year Performance			1,391,949	21,076,895	NA	NA	80,648	1,097,452

Figure 2.5. Performance of the gaining group.

Three Year Labor Performance

New Programs & Other

Quality Mgmt

	Unit of Service	Volume	Total Labor		Per Unit		Productivity Change	
			Hours	Wages	Hours	Wages	Hours	Wages
2000	Adj Discharges	16,808	0	0	0.0	0.00	0	0
2001	Adj Discharges	18,840	0	0	0.0	0.00	0	0
2002	Adj Discharges	20,441	8,820	208,326	0.4	10.19	0	0
Three Year Performance		56,089	8,820	208,326	0.2	3.71	0	0

Senior Health

	Unit of Service	Volume	Hours	Wages	Hours	Wages	Hours	Wages
2000	Visits	0	0	0	0.0	0.00	0	0
2001	Visits	1,202	3,505	60,223	2.9	50.10	0	0
2002	Visits	2,404	7,079	122,512	2.9	50.96	(69)	(1,194)
Three Year Performance		3,606	10,584	182,735	2.9	50.68	(69)	(1,194)

Drug Rehab

	Unit of Service	Volume	Hours	Wages	Hours	Wages	Hours	Wages
2000	Visits	0	0	0	0.0	0.00	0	0
2001	Visits	0	0	0	0.0	0.00	0	0
2002	Visits	2,582	7,079	122,512	2.7	47.45	0	0
Three Year Performance		2,582	7,079	122,512	2.7	47.45	0	0

(continued)

Three Year Labor Performance

		Unit of Service	Volume	Total Labor		Per Unit		Productivity Change	
				Hours	Wages	Hours	Wages	Hours	Wages
Respir Therapy	2000	RVUs	0	0	0	0.0	0.00	0	0
	2001	RVUs	60,839	16,077	275,816	0.3	4.53	0	0
	2002	RVUs	413,376	109,311	1,872,803	0.3	4.53	(74)	(1,275)
	Three Year Performance		474,215	125,388	2,148,619	0.3	4.53	(74)	(1,275)
Sleep Lab	2000	Visits	0	0	0	0.0	0.00	0	0
	2001	Visits	0	0	0	0.0	0.00	0	0
	2002	Visits	153	4,636	78,165	30.3	510.88	0	0
	Three Year Performance		153	4,636	78,165	30.3	510.88	0	0
Clinical Testing	2000	Contact Hours	0	0	0	0.0	0.00	0	0
	2001	Contact Hours	1,020	1,900	56,003	1.9	54.90	0	0
	2002	Contact Hours	2,331	3,440	110,432	1.5	47.38	902	28,958
	Three Year Performance		3,351	5,340	166,435	1.6	49.67	902	28,958
Total	2000			0	0	NA	NA	0	0
	2001			21,482	392,042	NA	NA	0	0
	2002			140,365	2,514,750	NA	NA	759	26,489
	Three Year Performance			161,847	2,906,792	NA	NA	759	26,489

Figure 2.6. Performance of the new programs and other group.

Generally, one quarter to one third of departments will place in the first group, Losing Ground. This category is of particular interest. The object of the analysis is to assess what it means to the organization if departments in the losing ground group returned to the standard of performance they had reached in the past (see Figure 2.3). The fourth group, New Programs and Other, is used to exclude start-ups and unusual departments from the analysis. New programs have not had sufficient time to establish stable patient volumes, much less staff in relation to workload (see Figure 2.6). "Other" might include grant or temporary programs where cost cutting is not an objective.

The second category, Holding Steady, is reserved for those departments with relatively little change over 3 years (see Figure 2.4). Depending on the numbers of each department, this group would generally be treated similarly to the third category, Gaining. If large productivity losses have occurred in certain years, however, such departments would be candidates for improvement.

The third category, Gaining, highlights departments that are more efficient now than in the past. It is important to inquire why this is the case. If this year's budget puts them at a higher standard of performance, it is sensible to request of managers that they just stick with the current budget. If their year-to-date actual productivity is better than ever, then asking them to maintain current performance is all that is required of them (see Figure 2.5). Figures 2.3–2.6 are condensed versions of what the whole report would look like.

For some people, rows and columns of figures fail to drive the point home. These people may represent a sizable portion of the executive and managerial audience, particularly if they have no financial training. It is constructive to graph the results. There are two ways of presenting the results of the analysis. Both methods should be used. The first chart would be a bar chart that separates the "gainers" from the "losers," taken straight from the analysis presented previously (see Figure 2.7). Breaking the groups apart like this illustrates the composition of historical productivity. Although some departments improved, some did not.

The second chart would be a bar chart that illustrates the Pareto Principle (or the "80/20" rule) applied to total savings (see Figure 2.8). This would show how most of the savings are concentrated in a few departments, with the rest distributed in smaller portions throughout the rest of the organization.

These sorts of graphs resonate with a number of department managers, who may already suspect that some kind of subsidy may be occurring at their expense. The unfairness of this situation is finally proven. If the whole organization is illustrated without any department identifiers, these graphs make their meaning clear without drawing unnecessary and undesirable attention to any manager or department. An objectionable and expensive hidden subsidy

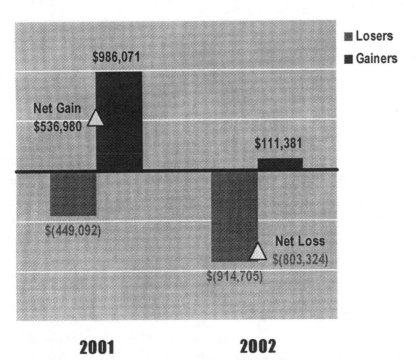

Figure 2.7. Composition of hospital productivity. Net gain of $536,980 in 2001 versus net loss of $803,324 in 2002 composed of *losers* and *gainers*.

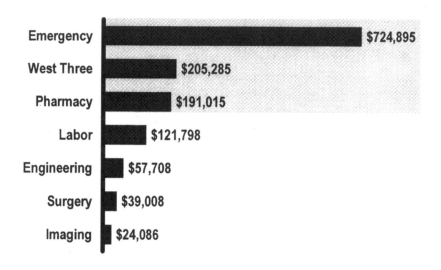

Figure 2.8. An example of the Pareto Principle (also called the 80/20 Rule). The top three departments represent 82% of total opportunity.

is occurring, and the organization is going to set it right. This puts things on a positive note.

The results should also be presented in terms of meeting important organization strategic and financial goals. Nearly every health care organization has a "mission statement," an expression of its core values. These mission statements often express the organization's commitment to efficiency and effectiveness, caring for patients regardless of ability to pay, and a pledge to provide the best-trained staff and technology to the public. Most organizations also have a strategic plan, one of whose pillars is financial strength. Now is the time to relate productivity to the organization's mission and strategy (please refer to Chapter 3 for further discussion of this topic).

How Many Years Are Best for the Analysis?

The right period of time for the analysis depends on several factors unique to the organization generally and to the departments specifically. Generally, the farther back the analysis goes, the greater the potential opportunity, especially if productivity has been sliding for several years. Going back more than 3 years, however, can pose significant challenges—different managers, processes, and functions, if present, make a more difficult analysis and may compromise acceptance. Three years is generally recent enough that, in the majority of cases, there has been no change in function and no real change in how department work is done. Even more important, there likely has been no change in department management. The options are these:

> "THE FARTHER BACK YOU CAN LOOK, THE FARTHER FORWARD YOU ARE LIKELY TO SEE."
>
> —WINSTON CHURCHILL

- Choose a period of 3 years for all departments. *Advantages:* simplicity and uniformity, perception of "fairness" since everyone is treated the same, no problems of being singled out, easier analysis, and better acceptance. *Disadvantages:* might miss productivity opportunities that may be difficult to capture later.

- Choose individual periods for every department. *Advantages:* capture the best productivity opportunities for each department, maximizing savings for the organization. *Disadvantages:* the "fairness" question.

Ultimately, the decision of which choice to make depends as much on politics as analysis. Whatever the choice, *taking action* is what matters most.

What to Expect

Without doing the analysis, it is difficult to guess at outcomes. So much depends on what the organization has done in the past; the various labor saving initiatives it may have undertaken, and whether there were significant and lasting results. In addition, often without anyone realizing it, the budget process tends to compound any labor problems over successive years. Managers request additions to their labor budgets, which, when granted, become the new base for the following year's budget. If managers happen to exceed their budgets, the excess can also become built into next year's budget.

Nevertheless, people want to know what to expect, so here is a reasonable expectation: at a medium-size hospital of about 250 beds, the savings opportunity should be about $2 million per year. Counting nonproductive time (vacation, sick, holiday) and benefits, the total should come to at least $2.6 million. This figure would be tempered (or stepped up) by any initiatives the organization has already undertaken. The savings tend to add up quickly because the whole organization is under the microscope, and the analysis looks for the best productivity ratios over several years for each department. If the hospital is twice as big (at 500 beds) it should expect to find double that amount, or more than $5 million. If the hospital is part of a 10-hospital system of 300-bed hospitals, and all of them are going through this productivity program, it would be reasonable to expect almost $3 million per facility multiplied by 10, or about $30 million.

Best of all, this is just the first plank on the road to better productivity. The program adjusts selected departments to similar staffing ratios that they had several years' back, in line with current volume. It does not, however, specify where departments should be in terms of their industry peers. Nor does the program specify where the organization must set its staffing to match its revenues. If the organization did not have nationally recognized productivity several years ago, as is very likely, a program of incentives will help take it there, as discussed in Chapter 5.

After the Analysis

It is relatively straightforward to analyze the data, assess the situation, and make a recommendation on realistic productivity targets. It is somewhat more complex to execute a rational plan and realize the expected results. As with any other initiative involving significant change while calling for widespread cooperation, three things must occur in sequence:

1. Managers and executives must be sold on the program to gain their commitment and resolve to follow through.

Eric is the radiology manager at Portland General. Eric's experience with budgets and productivity at other hospitals makes him apprehensive about the whole process that Portland General is going through. His department has gone through many changes. The number and mix of tests that are done are quite different now from a few years ago, since MRI has been added and CT has been expanded. The department has a weighting for each type of test it does, but no one had validated this since the last radiology manager set it up. Eric wants to make sure he gets this across to the people doing the analysis—and hopes they will listen.

---

2. The productivity system must be implemented in an orderly and methodical manner.

3. There must be intensive monitoring and protocols so the organization does not return to its old ways.

Chapters 3, 4, and 5 describe how this can be done.

Translating the Analysis into Standards

Although it can be hard to foresee what organizations might run into because every organization's culture is unique, sentiments are apt to be running high with any productivity plan. It is worth anticipating now so that the organization can deal with them. Some may complain that the plan will not work, and the task is to listen patiently for the *valid* objections. Remember that the goal is to *reclaim* lost productivity. By grounding the analysis and action plan firmly in history, it is highly realistic. The program does not involve an impossible series of "stretch goals." Rather, it recaptures that which had already been accomplished, reapplied to today's volumes.

Once the analysis is prepared, each of the department managers should be met with individually and their departmental results discussed. The goal is to secure managers' cooperation and have them accept history as a staffing guide. This step requires special adroitness. Managers may feel threatened and may adopt a defensive posture. The analysis should be used to talk openly about operations and productivity, not exploited as an indictment of past misdeeds. Cooperation, not confrontation, is called for.

- If current performance (defined as hours and perhaps cost per unit of service), is superior to that of the past, current productivity should be the starting point. For these departments, the task is relatively easy: request that they maintain current performance.

- If the current budget places a department at the peak of its historical productivity, the budget can serve as the frame of reference. If the budget appears realistic, the current budget would suffice.

- If historical productivity was better than it is now, history should be used.

Ideally, the analysis could be translated directly into productivity standards, but details about department operations may not be reflected in the analysis. Numbers may not tell the whole story. The presumption is that past performance should be replicable, but it is not certain. What makes the difference is a working knowledge of the department, its operations, its goals, and any other issues that should be considered prior to setting a standard.

This important phase allows proper consideration of individual circumstances before arriving at a realistic, mutually agreeable productivity standard. That is why individual, private meetings with the department managers are vital to lasting success. Both parties in the negotiation should come away with an agreement that is satisfactory to both. The negotiator wants to achieve the maximum savings possible, but the department manager wants something in return for the effort required. Both parties should be prepared to offer a little to achieve the desired outcome. As explained in Chapter 3, much will be offered to the department managers.

There Are No Shortcuts

Rapid execution and decisive action appear impressive. Realistic savings opportunities mixed with an urgent need for money would seem to dictate a swift course of action. Unfortunately, haste makes waste. If speed were the only concern, the organization could achieve its savings tomorrow with a layoff. After all the upheaval and dislocation, it would be doomed to see short-term gains erode and the organization return to where it started. Would it not be better to do it right the first time and not repeat mistakes of the past? The bulk of the effort and time involved in achieving superior productivity should be devoted to implementation, monitoring, incentives, consequences, and formulating new procedures to capture and build on what has been accomplished. That takes time and a little patience. The initial analysis is just the starting point.

Owing to productivity's importance in daily operations, managers may desire a series of meetings. Because of the time demands of numerous meetings, it might prove tempting to dispense with individual meetings in favor of larger, more efficient group presentations. The problem is that while a group presentation is efficient at imparting information, it is primarily a one-way information vehicle. The presenter can impart the program's goals and objectives, but cannot get much meaningful response from the group. People tend not to ask certain questions in public that they will in private, questions that would yield information critical to the ultimate success of the endeavor. Sharing personal information, or not grasping the information presented, may be embarrassing or impolite in public. The peculiar quietness familiar to any public speaker should not be taken as a sign of widespread agreement. Personal meetings and conversations help to overcome resistance and explain the organization's goals and the manager's role. They provide an opportunity to learn more about a manager's operation and consider his or her unique circumstances. The organization must understand and respond to all of its manager's questions and concerns. Only private meetings with department managers will accomplish this. The time spent with each manager will be well invested in producing a better outcome on implementation.

Sometimes speed is achieved at the cost of understanding, commitment, and lasting results. In the pressure for speed, it is all too easy to end up just being hasty. Anything that gets in the way of lasting results must be avoided.

Do You Need Outside Help?

It can be quite uncomfortable for a long-time member of the administrative staff to find him- or herself in the unpopular position of extracting savings from fellow managers, numbering among them colleagues and friends. Conflicts over priorities and roles can translate to rough going for a staff member.

It is critical that the organization be properly positioned to nurture this program through the first 6 months until it is well established and working smoothly. After this time, the new arrangement will become entrenched as a normal part of company culture. If the attempt is abandoned prematurely, the next initiative will lack credibility and will be that much harder to achieve. For these reasons, the organization should seriously consider hiring an outside expert to conduct the project from beginning to end. If hiring a consultant, it is best to pair him or her with an experienced and respected member of the finance or management engineering staff. This facilitates cross-training and fills in the gaps that any outsider will have about the inner workings of the health care organization.

Inevitably, there will be some problems and exceptions. By hiring a consultant to follow through from conception to implementation and monitoring, a powerful signal may be sent throughout the organization that the new productivity program is not the *fad du jour,* not something that will blow over, but standard operating procedure from now on. If there is, however, someone on staff with special expertise in matters of productivity who possesses sufficient objectivity, then such a person might well lead the project. Sufficient time must be allotted so that the undertaking receives the necessary amount of attention and priority it must have.

Executive Commitment

If executives have mixed feelings about pursuing this standards project, it is doomed to fail, no matter how brilliant and compelling the analysis, no matter how well orchestrated the implementation. If the will to succeed is lacking at the top, it simply will not happen. Department managers can readily sense whether the administration is entirely behind the endeavor; internal dissension might provide them an escape route. The key to making this program work and having a rewarding experience comes down to a complete, certain, no-reservations commitment to pursue success. The executive role in the productivity program is fully discussed in Chapters 3 and 5, which deal with implementation, incentives, and consequences.

How Long Will This Take?

A medium-size organization will need about 3 months to complete the analytical process, engage the managers, and begin implementation. If multiple facilities are involved, it is best to have several individuals or small groups conduct the meetings in parallel with the other campuses. This will save time and keep the project moving ahead at the same pace for all.

It is a considerable advantage to have the same individual or small group conduct all manager meetings within the same facility.

This produces consistency and better learning, albeit at a small sacrifice of speed. If the organization does not face imminent bankruptcy, it should be willing to trade some speed for greater accuracy and a more profitable outcome. Three months is not a lot of time to achieve something so important. The emphasis has to be on a successful result because a lot is on the line, both culturally and economically. Managers will appreciate the time and consideration given them at this stage. The extra time is critical for gaining manager commitment.

Managing for Change

It has already been strongly recommended that managers be met individually and privately to hear their concerns and take into account the particulars of their operations. At this point, managers will likely be concerned as to what use the analysis will be put, what will be expected of them, and whether they will feel comfortable in the new business environment and remain committed. Fear of the unknown is always a factor lurking in any big program of change, possibly driven by the manager's experience of what went on before.

Executives can do a lot to overcome these qualms by being completely open and honest with their managers. They would do well to explain the complete program that they are putting the organization through: its necessity, its methods, and its outcomes. Executives need to elaborate what the new management principles will mean to the department managers as they go through the program. They need to be available for open discussion at any time.

Patient Type	Patient Days 2001	2002	Patient Mix 2001	2002	Hours per Unit 2001	2002
Medical/Surgical	8,500	7,000	85%	70%	9.5	9.5
Oncology	1,500	3,000	15%	30%	12.0	12.0
Total	10,000	10,000	100%	100%	9.9	10.3

Figure 2.9. Accounting for changing service mix.

Above all, they need to support the program without reservations, demonstrating sheer leadership by emphasizing the task that they themselves face. Executives must impart to their managers the conviction that everyone will be up to the undertaking, emphasizing that no one will be allowed unwittingly to fail, that all the support needed will be provided to succeed.

Much has been written in management books about how difficult it can be to change company culture and the long years it can take to achieve real change. True, people will often resist change and attempt to disrupt the best-laid plans. There is also, however, literature to demonstrate that a complete, coherent program implemented in the briefest possible time has the best possible chance of success. If the basic operating rules of the organization change, then corresponding attitudes and behaviors will follow as a natural result. To do the reverse—attempt to change attitudes and then change the operating rules—is to invite all but certain failure. Talking about change for an extended time is sufficient to induce needless apprehension all by itself. It is much better to make the changes required and then help people along. The approach in this book to address such issues is threefold:

1.   Describe the changes to the practice of productivity management throughout the organization as completely and fully as possible at the commencement of the program, but not too far in advance. People have a right to know what is coming, and there is no need to be secretive.

	Patient Days		Patient Mix		Total Hours		Hours per Unit	
	2001	2002	2001	2002	2001	2002	2001	2002
Medical/Surgical	8,500	7,000	85%	70%	80,750	66,500	9.5	9.5
Oncology	1,500	3,000	15%	30%	18,000	36,000	12.0	12.0
Total	10,000	10,000	100%	100%	98,750	102,500	9.9	10.3
Weighted Days	8,229	8,542	NA	NA	98,750	102,500	12.0	12.0

Figure 2.10.   Weighting multiple patient types.

2. Emphasize the benefits to the organization and to the individual manager that the program entails. As outlined in Chapters 3–5, these include new manager authority and prerogatives; realistic labor standards, not "stretch" targets; simplified, understandable reporting; and meaningful incentives to exceed the minimum.

3. Stress that this is not an impossible task and that successful productivity management is well within the capacity of every manager in the organization. Underline that the organization is committed to the program and will make it happen. Such conviction inspires confidence.

Comparing Apples and Oranges

A department that has altered its basic function or services presents a valid challenge to using historical performance as a guide to setting standards. It is as if the old department is no more. In such cases, productivity standards can still be created using current performance. Although this may have little impact now, it will help prevent productivity losses in the future. A similar situation arises in newly created departments, and those that are relatively new. Current productivity and budgets can be used to develop productivity standards in new departments.

In some cases, history can still be useful even if there has been a functional change in the department. Suppose, for illustration, a nursing unit accepted two patient types last year, and this year the mix has changed in favor of a higher proportion of the more acute type. In other words, last year the unit had a different patient mix than this year, and it is likely to continue shifting over time. In this example, a weighting scheme can be used to make use of the department's history. An in-house acuity measure can be established, with the manager's agreement, applicable to this particular unit. This weighting scheme constitutes a productivity standard by patient type. Whenever the patient mix shifts, multiple standards by patient type account for the new patient mix. This allows the organization to evaluate historical department productivity and factors out the effect of changing service mix in performance monitoring, an important consideration for accuracy and fairness.

Illustration: Accounting for Changing Service or Patient Mix

In the example in Figure 2.9, for simplicity, the total number of patients is the same from one year to the next, but the patient mix is not. The patient mix was 85% medical/surgical in 2001 and 70% in 2002, while oncology patients were 15% and 30%, respectively. By way of interviews and supporting data, the analyst calculates that each medical/surgical patient takes 9.5 hours worked per patient day, and oncology patients get 12.0 hours worked per patient day. These values should be the same for both years. In 2001, productivity was 9.9 hours worked per patient day for the whole department. In 2002, as the department's patient mix changed, the average for the department was 10.3 hours worked per patient day.

The analytical task is to make sure that when hours worked per patient day for each patient type are multiplied by their respective volumes, the total agrees with the department's total worked hours. No matter how the manager wants to account for different patient types, the actual hours per patient day for each patient type must be equal for both years. Two labor standards will be used for this department, 9.5 for medical/surgical, and 12.0 for oncology. From Figure 2.7, the department is equivalent in productivity from one year to the next, even though hours worked per patient day rose from 9.9 to 10.3, solely due to the changing patient mix. It would be grossly unfair to punish the manager for apparently bad performance, when, in fact, nothing is wrong.

Simple patient days as a workload statistic will not work very well for the department, since different patient days require different amounts of labor. Yet, the goal is to produce a single unit of service as a calculation for productivity. How can this be done? The service mix issue can be dealt with by adjusting "raw" patient days into a single workload statistic, *weighted patient days*. A medical/surgical patient day would have a different weight than an oncology patient day. Weighted patient days, as the unit of service, will account for any changes in patient mix automatically. Taking the previous illustration a step farther, weighted patient days can be calculated as seen in Figure 2.10.

Note that hours per weighted patient day are 12.0 for both years, exactly the result wanted because true productivity is really the same for both years. The department can use more patient types than were used here. Some ancillary units may have 10 or even 20 different labor values to match the number of procedures offered. Whatever the number of patient categories used, the general idea remains the same. The analyst assigns a realistic labor value for each patient type, and then multiplies the labor value by the number of patients in each category to ensure that total hours are equal to what the department actually used. If they are not equal, he assigns slightly different hours per unit of service to each patient type until the hours tie out. These unit values are used to weight patient days to derive a single labor standard for the department that automatically accounts for the proportion of different patients on the unit.

Any unit that has significant numbers of different types of patients requiring different treatments, or standards of care that vary for each patient type or treatment, can use this method. Many inpatient-nursing units, for example, provide care for "observation" patients who spend the day on the unit and require service, but who miss the midnight census and the official workload count. Many ancillary patient care departments commonly use different labor values by type of procedure. Of course, this assumes that department staff are actually spending different amounts of time for each patient type on the unit. Although the weighting of patient days factors out any changes in the service mix, the unit would still actually be staffed so that each type of patient receives the appropriate planned hours of care.

Tracking days or procedures by patient type is not a cumbersome task if the charge master is used, or some other automated way of reporting patient types is employed. For the analyst, manager, and executive, it simplifies monitoring as well, because it factors out the productivity impact of varying patient types. That makes it easier to spot trends that need corrective action, separating real problems from those that are not.

Internal Benchmarking

In larger organizations, multiple units of the same type may care for similar types of patients. In addition, multicampus systems often have similar units amongst their various facilities. These offer an opportunity to benchmark *internally* with the best performer, using its standard of performance for other units of its type. First, a note of caution is in order.

Operations must be compared for anything unique among the units. The most efficient department might, for example, owe its performance to its larger size. In that case, combining several smaller departments may duplicate the conditions, and thus the efficiency, of the best performer. A financial analysis would reveal whether this is worthwhile, given the costs of any remodeling and reorganizing.

Although this entails a comparison outside the unit, it is considerably short of searching for best-demonstrated practice anywhere it exists in the country—or even outside the health care industry. The tough part of *external benchmarking*—equating different patients, medical practices, traditions, workload counting, and tasks—is minimized to the point where it might be a good idea to take up this kind of intra-organization, internal benchmarking at the outset. Middle management resistance will certainly be less than what would be encountered when going outside the organization or system. On the other hand, if internal benchmarking is a hindrance in getting the rest of the program off to a good start, it can be pursued later. In any case, it may be a very good way to capture "best practice" within the hospital's walls.

SUMMARY

Control over labor costs—the largest single category of expense—can be regained by developing sound labor standards. Drawing from each department's history, standards are the result of careful negotiation supported by hard data. Effective standards mean defining what the organization expects of its managers. By comparing each department's past performance to its current efficiency, slipping productivity can be reversed. History serves as a very accurate guide to the organization's potential for productivity improvement.

Workload measures, or "units of service," should be assigned for every department. The unit of service is a measure of a department's main output, not its inputs. Department managers must agree that their unit of service is appropriate. If not, other measures should be substituted until agreement is reached. Combining workload with hours and salaries determines each department's productivity loss or gain for several years. The results reveal the savings each department could achieve by operating at a better standard of performance.

The number of years to use in the analysis depends on factors unique to the organization. Generally, the farther back the analysis goes, the greater the potential opportunity. Going back more than 3 years, however, may compromise acceptance. Three years is generally recent enough that there has been no change in function or process.

Once the analysis is prepared, each of the department managers should be met with individually. Details about department operations that are not reflected in the analysis need to be taken into account. This important phase allows proper consideration of individual circumstances before arriving at a realistic, mutually agreeable productivity standard.

After the analysis, managers and executives should be sold on the program to gain their commitment and resolve, the productivity system should be implemented methodically, and there ought to be extensive follow through so the organization does not return to its old ways. Shortcuts in the process are to be avoided. It may be best to hire an outside expert to manage the project if an insider with expertise and sufficient time cannot be found. A medium-sized organization will take about 3 months to go through the analytical process, engage the managers, and begin implementation.

At this point, managers will likely be concerned as to what use the analysis will be put, what will be expected of them, and whether they will feel comfortable and remain committed in the new business environment. Executives can do a lot to overcome these qualms and concerns by being completely open and honest with their managers.

In larger organizations and systems, there may be an opportunity to benchmark internally with similar departments. Before doing this, operations should be compared for anything unique among the units. If this comparison does not present an obstacle and the units are functionally comparable, then "internal benchmarking" might be done right away. If not, it should be saved for a later project.

C•H•A•P•T•E•R 3

IMPLEMENTATION

Realistic standards offer the best means to improve and maintain productivity. Staffing standards must be soundly devised and correctly implemented if they are to work as intended. There are, however, certain core productivity concepts and management problems that must be resolved before reporting and monitoring tools are designed.

Workable standards are simple, easily understood, and widely accepted as valid and practical. Alas, conventional productivity measurement systems actually hinder, not help, this mission. Perhaps the most important factor for success, however, is not the monitoring system but the courage to enforce standards uniformly and equitably throughout the organization. That comes far ahead of any concern for mathematical precision in measurements.

Difficult as it may be to delegate to their managers, executives should remove themselves from basic productivity decisions. By delegating authority and providing a firm set of realistic standards to each department manager, any potential abuses of power can be circumvented. Then, department managers can focus on the improvement process and executives can concentrate on outcome.

This book makes the case that department managers can, and should, control their own department's productivity, with all of the necessary power to act on their own authority—provided they act within their standards. This chapter provides the operating framework for doing just that. The plan calls for new organizational rules to govern productivity management. The rules cover manager authority and responsibility, changes to standards, and executive oversight and management.

"I CAN GIVE YOU A SIX-WORD FORMULA FOR SUCCESS: THINK THINGS THROUGH, THEN FOLLOW THROUGH."
—EDDIE RICKENBACKER

Fixed and Variable: Fact or Fiction?

Productivity measurement systems divide labor hours and costs into *variable* and *fixed* categories, meaning that staffing varies with workload volume, or it does not. The purpose of splitting staff into variable and fixed divisions comes from the idea that with growth in volume, fewer people need to be hired if departments have a fixed portion that does not increase with work volume. As volume decreases, however, there is less need to flex down, again due to the fixed component of the department. A department classified as 50% fixed and 50% variable, for example, would grow by only 5% if volume rose 10% ($50\% \times 10\% = 5\%$). The same department would shrink by only 5% when presented with a 10% reduction in volume.

The fixed/variable cost theory says that as the organization grows, it becomes more efficient; if the organization shrinks, it becomes less efficient. On the surface, this makes some sense, in that a larger organization should be better able to absorb hypothetically fixed administration costs, spreading them over a larger base. This implies some fixed level of administrative costs that is not related to the size of the patient base. These fixed costs would be found in such departments as housekeeping, billing, medical records, coding, financial planning and budgeting, personnel, marketing and public relations, and information systems. If these departments did not grow with the organization, then large organizations and systems should have the same fixed overhead load as small organizations. Large facilities, and especially hospital systems, should be enormously more efficient and cost-effective than their smaller counterparts.

The problem is that administrative costs are not fixed. Virtually all of these functions are related in some way to the size of the organization, its patient load, the number and types of services it offers, and the number of new services it plans to introduce into its market. In fact, as the organization grows, administrative and other overhead labor costs are likely to grow even faster, making them not just variable, but *super-variable,* growing faster than the patient base. It is simply not true that an organization has a certain amount of fixed cost regardless of its size. Any large organization will have much more administrative cost than an organization half or a quarter its size. Throughout the industry, especially in the past few years, supposedly fixed administrative and support functions have at least kept pace with organization growth, often exceeding it.

Mechanics of Fixed/Variable Splitting

The measurement of the fixed component within the variable (mostly clinical) departments is no easy task. Usually this involves management engineers running around to the departments and inquiring about "fixed" positions such as manager, supervisor, charge nurse, lead technician, and so on. Everyone else is deemed to have a direct relation to workload and is designated "variable." Some jobs are actually split within themselves. A certain position might, for example, be classified as 80% variable and 20% fixed. Other positions in the same department might be classified as 100% variable, or 50% variable, or 100% fixed. A productivity report based on such complex calculations would come to the manager as a complete surprise. This is not a desirable situation.

Because staffing and workload are likely to be fluid over time, accuracy demands that this process be repeated at least annually. Owing to time and resource constraints, however, this may be done much more infrequently. As the composition of most departments will almost certainly change over time, the original measurements will become invalid.

Notwithstanding the above, these are merely difficulties in measurement and calculation, primarily mechanical and cyclical in nature, overcome with the expenditure of some time and money. Such would be a small price to pay if it were worth it, but time and money are not the main objections to fixed/variable department splitting.

Fixed and Variable within the Department

Broadly speaking, the whole concept of "fixed" staff is largely a myth wrapped around a kernel of truth. Although it has validity over short time spans, it falls apart over the course of a year or longer. It may be true that hiring fixed employees lags changes in volume, but it keeps pace with variable employee hiring soon enough. In fact, virtually the only jobs that do not increase with workload are those that have no obvious work volume driver, something measurable linked to the amount of work to be done. Perhaps the CEO or CFO fits this description, but even then, this person is likely to hire assistants when he or she cannot cope with extra work, and these assistants are often vice presidents or chief operating officers. Although department managers as a class are not likely to grow much in number, the head count of supervisors and assistants supporting them certainly will. "Variable" employees may follow a more smoothly graduated path to accommodate workload changes, but there is no real difference between the groups. In most cases, the distinction between fixed and variable is artificial. Even if the belief in fixed costs were accurate in the short term, everything is variable over the long term (a year or more), including wholly "fixed" departments, those with no variable component at all.

The experience with fixed and variable splitting within the same department is that such arrangements are confusing and poorly understood by department managers. It introduces unnecessary complexity and confusion, defeating the whole purpose of having a productivity system in the first place. This can be verified easily enough by simply asking managers to explain the conceptual foundation of the system currently in use. Next, they can be asked to explain the productivity calculations for their own department. The results are usually quite revealing. Few managers are likely fluent enough in management engineering to understand their own system, and no amount of educational seminars or "brown bag" educational lunches seems to make the slightest difference. That is the first indication of a major problem: no one understands it. Without understanding and acceptance, it would be unreasonable to expect such a productivity management system to produce anything of significant or lasting value.

Illustration

A nursing unit has 22 FTEs, of which two are fixed: manager and supervisor. The span of control is 20:2, or 10:1. Suppose the organization recruits new doctors, they bring in more patients, and the department hires 10 new people to care for the additional patients. The department now has 32 FTEs, but it still has the same two fixed staff. The manager and supervisor now manage 30 employees for a 15:1 span of control.

Will managing 50% more employees mean anything to the workload of the manager and supervisor? It certainly will. Once this situation goes on for any length of time, the manager will undoubtedly observe that his or her workload and that of the supervisor is much greater than before. The manager will take the first opportunity to plead for more fixed staff: another supervisor perhaps, a clerk, and so on. Budgeting season is a convenient time to bring the department back into balance, and in due course, the manager will almost certainly receive permission to increase the fixed staff contingent. In effect, this makes fixed staff variable.

Organizations do adjust the fixed component of their labor standards periodically when conditions warrant. That is perfectly reasonable. What are those conditions? Many reasons might be offered, but the most common by far is an increase in employees to manage! This is a familiar scenario; one repeated so commonly as to form the following rule:

> Fixed staff varies with variable staff.
> Variable staff varies with volume.
> Therefore,
> Fixed staff varies with volume.

Scott runs the patient billing department. The department has billers, coders, and collectors on a variable standard, and others—managers supervisors, secretarial—are part of the "fixed" staff. As the hospital has grown, Scott has added many more billers, coders, and collectors over the last few years. More people to supervise impose a greater administrative load for each fixed staff member to handle. He can hardly keep up with employee reviews, new hiring, and the ongoing training he is committed to providing. He would like to "catch-up" by hiring several new fixed supervisors and secretaries to keep his department in the proper balance. If permission is denied or delayed, he will have to warn the CFO that receivables may rise and cash balances may decline.

The route to more fixed staff may be a jagged line. This is also known as "step-variable," meaning that fixed staff tends to increase in irregular spurts, not smoothly with patient volume. Over time, it all leads to the same place anyway.

It is suggested that this hypothetical department cannot maintain a 15:1 span of control? In fact, it might be possible, but it might not. In any case, this is not the time to engage in department restructuring. The proper place and time to address this is through "internal benchmarking," analyzing spans of control throughout the organization to see what might be done in terms of management restructuring. In the meantime, the reality is that managers who can show increased spans of control will normally get some extra administrative help to manage a larger department.

When they have the option, managers generally prefer to add fixed staff over variable specifically to escape a direct link to workload. This allows them to add staff faster than workload volume by itself would justify, simply because fixed staff by definition is not variable with workload. A manager can add staff for new, supposedly "fixed" functions, without regard to overall department workload. This translates to an increase in standard, and that is why it is possible to meet standard every year in a conventional productivity system even while incurring more total hours per unit of service. Such a situation represents slipping productivity.

Adjusting standards to add more fixed staff is a serious problem that is addressed later in this chapter (see Rules for Changing Standards). Often accomplished during budget season, it also takes place during the year by way of the same hiring approval procedures that are supposed to prevent this from happening, but actually promote it. The analysis from Chapter 2 purposely ignores any distinction between fixed and variable jobs for this very reason, shining the spotlight on deteriorating productivity. The analysis simply compared total input to total output, so that valuable conclusions could be drawn. Had the traditional fixed/variable split been preserved, the opportunity would be largely missed.

Organizations seem to have created a serious rut from which there is no escape. Executives discuss, meet, plead, cajole, worry, and threaten, all to no avail—fussing about with a great deal of activity but rooted to the same spot.

Don't Shield Managers from Managing

Administration should get out of the business of determining fixed from variable costs. It is best to leave the task to department managers and not interfere with the proper exercise of good department management. If senior management attempts to exercise control, they will probably do a mediocre job of it, and managers will be encouraged to abdicate their responsibility. That greatly explains the nature of the problem.

Conventional productivity systems shield managers from having to make difficult choices when business conditions demand action. The larger the fixed component in a department, the more this is true. The fixed component prevents making any changes to at least that part of the department; after all, it is fixed. This is most unfortunate, for managers should always be adjusting their staffing with workload, they should not be saved from having to carry out this vital task. If management decisions are avoided early on, over time and given a sufficient downturn in business, more drastic measures such as layoffs, freezes, and across-the-board cuts are inevitable. Desperate measures like these thrust havoc on individuals and damage company culture. Perhaps more important, emergency, sweeping action usually proves to be purely short term. As the real problems are not addressed, irregular and drastic "corrections" must be repeated. Temporary emergency and financial crises become more or less permanent, and management loses control over one of its most basic charges.

Staffing must be continually adjusted to new business conditions; if not gracefully, invisibly, and routinely, then erratically, publicly, and clumsily by the board. Someone will have to do it. Forced into this onerous role because of the organization's failure to push authority and responsibility down to the operating level, the board has no particular fondness for it, nor are they very good at it.

No one wants a productivity system to impede sound management. The worth of any productivity system that prevents managers from adapting steadily to new business conditions is highly questionable. Regardless of how a fixed/variable split looks on paper, real-world experience with fixed and variable splitting in the same department has led to unintended consequences that outweigh any hypothetical benefits.

THE NEW DEAL

The analysis from the last chapter uncovered genuine opportunities. What worked so well as an analytical tool can now be used as the foundation for developing productivity standards. Having finished the analysis and contended with current industry practices, a strong case can be made for a new system of straightforward concepts and principles, more in harmony with the way managers actually run their departments, making it highly effective for that reason alone.

Let Managers Manage

Managers are hired primarily for having strong technical expertise in their field and the ability to coordinate the work of others. Yet, managing scarce resources efficiently is also essential to the health care mission. Although the clinical mission is commonly well supported, the task of promoting efficiency is hampered when managers lack genuine responsibility. Department managers may have formal accountability, but in practice productivity decisions are usually assigned to executives or the finance department, leaving department managers with paper responsibility only. Unless this problem is addressed, such split responsibility makes it possible for department managers to evade their productivity standards.

Managing labor costs is a function of matching the right number of people to a given workload, employing the right kinds of skills required for the types of services provided. It is not particularly mysterious. Why should organizations complicate something that is uncomplicated?

Remember that the new standards discussed in Chapter 2 are crafted from the departments' own history so that impossible "stretch goals" are not being decreed without a viable way to achieve them. Managers can handle the responsibility.

Don't Take Testimony

Most organizations make hiring decisions by executive committee. Regardless of the specific arrangement, the process is similar. Department managers are brought before the committee to give "testimony" that sounds much like this: Staff is overworked, and patients are not getting quality care. The department has grown. There are more meetings to attend. A doctor has written a testimonial letter for the executive committee. The inescapable conclusion: They must have more people so that the organization can continue operating. More staff members will undoubtedly fix the problem. The committee considers the appeal and renders a decision.

More often than not, this lament is effective and the committee grants approval for the manager to hire. It becomes exceedingly difficult to separate emotions from facts and to decide a case strictly on its merits. The only person really in a position to know is the department manager, and so the committee generally goes along. Moreover, it feels good to give, to dole out rewards to the deserving while denying petitions from the unworthy. One can feel generous and powerful at the same time. Who can honestly say that he or she is not moved by emotion? In fact, many decisions come through emotional persuasion—it feels right, it pleases the requesting party, and people want to get along with each other. Taken individually, these are often "little" decisions that do not seem important enough on which to take a stand. Why risk saying no—especially when others seem to get theirs? A small decision here, a small decision there—what difference does that make to a large business?

Unfortunately, running a business by what feels right is not a sound long-term strategy. The problem is the testimonial process itself, placing authority and responsibility with a committee, not the manager in charge. The people at the best level to control productivity, department managers, do not bear ultimate responsibility. If the executive committee makes the decision, it, not the managers, bears responsibility for the outcome. That sets up the organization for a huge problem down the road, for the people actually doing the hiring are not involved in daily operations that are the core of productivity management. The people that are able to control productivity, department managers, have only paper responsibility at best, lacking genuine hiring authority. Managers have every incentive to staff up, without having to bear the consequences that the whole organization must face eventually.

The only way to avoid the trap of emotional decision making is to replace emotion-based decision making with explicit rules derived from rational principles by which to govern the organization's actions. Health care organizations urgently need to drive politics out of decisions by clearly articulating the new rules proposed later in this chapter and in Chapter 5.

The testimonial process actually trains department managers how to beg effectively and teaches executives how to bestow favors. The whole testimony and approval process should be abolished. This is no way to run a business.

Budget Discipline: Missing in Action

What happens during the actual approval process? Obtaining the proper signatures to commence hiring usually involves a committee of senior managers who, on hearing testimony, sign off on the hiring approval according to some protocol. Perhaps the protocol requires that one or two vice presidents outside of the requesting division furnish their signatures to obtain approval. Perhaps unanimous consent of the committee is needed. No matter how many signatories are required, the rationale is the same, as are the results. The premise is that the approval process provides a check against unregulated hiring because the requesting vice president has to convince one or more fellow vice presidents to agree to his or her petition.

The unintended consequence is to increase spending even more. In an effort to satisfy both parties, the actual agreement that is inevitably reached goes something like this: a vice president will agree to a hiring request if he or she can get similar approval for his or her own division. Because all divisions normally want to hire some people at any given time, an agreement is easily reached, and it results in double the hiring—"one for you, and one for me." That is the area of most common ground, and that is how deals are struck. Not only is it difficult to know if his own managers are short, it can be impossible for a vice president to evaluate whether another division really requires more people. One thing the vice president knows is that cost aside, his or her own division would run more easily and smoothly with extra staff, and his or her own division is the first priority. If other vice presidents feel the same about their divisions, so the reasoning goes, then they should be given the benefit of the doubt, too.

Outside the health care field, a similar process is at work in Congress. A certain member of Congress wants a federal project for his or her district to show the folks back home that he is doing something for the local economy, for instance. The project may be unimportant to other representatives who want to secure something for their own districts, yet the member of Congress must gain the support of his or her colleagues to get his bill passed. The solution is that each Congress member agrees to support the other, and then both can get what they want. Moreover, it is easy to strike such deals because they use other people's money. This *pork-barrel* spending inflates the cost of government.

Back at the health care organization, the president could exercise his or her veto authority, but using it would threaten his or her working relationships with the vice presidents. Again, there is the "knowledge problem," but this time it is even more acute. As much as a vice president outside the requesting party's division finds it difficult to evaluate the true need for additional staff, the president would have even more difficulty making such a judgment, being removed one step further from the chain of command. It is not possible to have a thorough working knowledge of each department at the level of the CEO, nor is that even the CEO's job.

The chain of events leading to a budget crisis is clear-cut. Spending approval resides with top management, but no senior manager is *individually* responsible for a budget crisis befalling the organization. Senior management is collectively responsible. Of what practical use is collective responsibility? When everyone is responsible, then no one is. Just as the country's president would find it difficult to effectively restrain spending, so too would the health care president find it tough to guide the organization back to a responsible path. The approval processes and the prevailing incentives lead in the opposite direction. This is how organizations find themselves drifting until they are forced to act.

Granting ultimate hiring authority to senior management unintentionally results in overspending. That is not a slam against the skills of senior managers at running their organizations. However talented, it is not realistic to expect some people to make correct decisions for others all of the time. Senior management concern is more appropriately devoted to strategic direction and departmental coordination. Overspending is a problem of knowledge and incentives. If these were aligned properly, the problem would be fixed. No refinement of the present system that leaves the problem of knowledge and incentives untouched can succeed.

Aristotle said, "Small mistakes in the beginning can lead to enormous errors in the end." Most crises take some time to build, growing one small step at a time. It is only because they are not recognized until later that they appear to have come suddenly from nowhere. A seemingly trivial decision now can have enormous consequences later. One new hire per week for a year can subtract $2.5 million from the bottom line, enough to plunge many organizations into loss.

Accountability: The Brave New World

Achieving superior productivity has nothing much to do with hardware or software, micromonitoring, flash reports, or detailed budgets. These things are top-down command and control concepts that have removed ultimate accountability from the department managers' shoulders, the exact opposite of what organizations require. No amount of budget policing can compensate for a lack of individual responsibility and accountability. If this fundamental issue is tackled successfully, everything else falls into place. If the organization pursues a course of increasing its centralized grip on department managers, it can expect purely temporary results, if that. Productivity is not about technology or monitoring, it is about management. Management makes the difference.

Individual Accountability

Beyond just measuring *things,* an effective productivity management system encourages personal responsibility for maintaining performance to standard. The hiring committee may incur a collective responsibility, but it lacks the specific operations experience and the daily working relationship with department staff that only the department manager could possibly have.

Accountability is a necessary building block for any large, effective organization. The alternative is micromanagement from the top. Such a system depends on those at the top having a comprehensive working knowledge of all employees, patients, and information concerning every aspect of the business, at every moment. As a practical matter, in a medium-size organization or bigger, this is impossible. Friedrich von Hayek, Nobel laureate, explained in his land mark *The Fatal Conceit: The Errors of Socialism* (University of Chicago Press, 1991) how these conditions could never be met, and that any system depending on all-inclusive knowledge by a few at the top could not be sustained. It is the core reason that socialist, centrally planned economies are inferior to free-market, decentralized economies. Central planning cannot efficiently tap into, nor can it make effective use of, the vast pool of knowledge that exists in every organization, much less an entire country.

Responsibility must be matched with authority or it is meaningless. To make the new productivity system work, individual responsibility must be instilled for maintaining performance to standard. Such responsibility properly belongs to the department manager. In the new scheme, vice presidents continue to be responsible for the performance of each department in their division, but the department manager is ultimately accountable—in the line of fire. For people to be both responsible and accountable, they must have the power to act. Responsibility without authority is a formula for failure, for if a person is held responsible for producing tangible results but has no authority to make the necessary changes, he or she is set up for frustration and failure. Logically, without operating authority no one can truly be held accountable. It is a paper responsibility, utterly unworkable. What is more, if a department manager lacks the authority to make change, it follows that others outside his or her department must be accountable. The problem is that those who have such authority do not have the close day-to-day operating knowledge necessary to make decisions on the fly as circumstances change.

When power and responsibility are vested in different people, a cycle can unwittingly be set up that virtually guarantees things will get out of hand eventually. Having power without responsibility can easily generate huge cost overruns. With its paper-thin margins, the health care industry can ill afford this. If some people make decisions for others, who are then held accountable, no one need bear the consequences of their actions. That is simply human nature at work, responding to the prevailing system of incentives. The solution is coupling authority with responsibility. Any productivity program that confers power to one person while conveying responsibility to another is doomed to failure. If things are really going to change for the better, then health care organizations have to strike at the core of the problem.

Why do department managers tend not to spend in a more frugal manner? After all, many of the same people are perfectly capable of balancing their personal expenditures with their income. The great majority of people do not write bad checks or get into credit trouble because conducting their affairs irresponsibly carries with it unwelcome consequences. Responsibility is learned by the natural consequences of the decisions they make every day. Why do they not exercise similar restraint in business? The answer is because they do not have to; the present management structure allows a fair degree of non-compliance, shifting blame to others, and offering various excuses—some statistical, some cultural. That will not do in the new regime. Compliance will not be an option, blame will not be entertained, and excuses—barring highly unusual, exceptional circumstances—will be eliminated. Let each manager know that his future depends largely on his own actions. That is what the new system of productivity management will accomplish for the organization where the old one failed.

The organization must push accountability for results on the department manager's shoulders. Although authority is traditionally vested in executives, no other management level will do. Executives have to be willing to loosen the reins a bit and relieve themselves of direct day-to-day management and productivity problems they face. *They have to learn to let their managers take charge.* Managers, in turn, require the authority to make the necessary changes to meet and exceed standards. Responsibility in the absence of power will not work.

Executive Accountability

Where does this leave the executives? Because vice presidents are responsible for the departments within their divisions, performance problems in any of their departments are theirs as well. In quarterly productivity reviews, averaging a division will be avoided because savings opportunities are buried in the averages. A divisional average would also compromise individual accountability because gains from the better performers would erase the losses of the worst performers, wiping out any consequences and the catalyst for improvement. Furthermore, a division is just a collection of departments, a chain of command. Some departments may be interrelated, and some are not. Be that as it may, the organization chart does not matter in the least. For supreme accountability, each department must stand on its own, on the same footing as all others.

> "DON'T BE AFRAID TO TAKE A BIG STEP IF ONE IS INDICATED; YOU CAN'T CROSS A CHASM IN TWO SMALL JUMPS."
> —DAVID LLOYD GEORGE

If vice presidents are going to be responsible for the performance of their divisions, in all fairness, they have to assume the same responsibility they are thrusting onto their managers. If executives are accountable for each of their departments, they too are responsible for each of their departments meeting standard. In fact, the greater one's rank and authority, the greater one's accountability ought to be. There is not one rule for "them" and another rule for "us." This is strongly positive because it builds considerable trust.

Although department managers have direct responsibility, by following the same rules, everyone pulls together.

That said, executive accountability is still of secondary concern. How to handle executive accountability will vary from place to place. On one hand, zero executive accountability will foster lack of initiative and concerns of unfairness that will permeate the organization. On the other hand, 100% accountability, although desirable in principle, must mean something different for the executive than for the manager. It would not be reasonable for a manager to be fired for the poor performance of just one of his or her departments. It would be entirely appropriate, however, for that executive to fix the situation or face the consequences of inaction. That may be demanding, but responsibility has to work up and down the ladder. The CEO is responsible for the performance of the entire organization and he or she should not hesitate to delegate some of that responsibility—and the authority that belongs with it—to the rest of the executive team.

Executives should concentrate on managing the outcome, not the process. The managers will be accountable for maintaining performance to standard; anything that interferes with their ability to act is an obstacle to be eliminated. With the new authority and accountability, the organization thus rids itself of any excuses for poor performance. From this line of reasoning, it is clear what needs to be done:

1. Abolish all senior manager approvals and sign-offs for hiring new people into the organization. For department managers to be completely accountable, they need the power to hire and fire whomever they see fit, on their own authority. No other approvals are necessary or desirable (reference checks, licensing requirements, and all of the normal hiring procedures still apply).

2. All hiring by department managers must fit within the productivity and cost standards for their departments, which will be carefully monitored (see Chapter 4).

3. Funding for new positions or new functions continue to need committee approval based on the merits of the case.

Whether hiring is for replacing departing employees, filling vacancies, or for additional volume, the reasons for hiring ought to be irrelevant to administration. As long as new hires fit within the confines of each department's productivity standards, administration ought to be pleased. How will administration know that is the case? Departments will be carefully monitored. If productivity standards are not met over the course of a quarter, the executive committee will step in (see Chapter 5 for the details).

In the new regime, with their new powers and new responsibilities, managers can hire up when volume increases, but they have to trim down when volume decreases. In practice, most managers will almost certainly not ride the peaks and troughs of normal volume fluctuations up and down too closely but seek a more stable middle ground. This strategy will serve them well. Like a bank account, the new system of extended performance reviews allows managers to "save" money when not presently needed against future circumstances when they might want to draw down on their "account." Rather than spending as fast as possible up to the limit allowed (the incentive of the current system), the new system encourages saving whenever possible, discarding the "use it or lose it" mentality. Managers never "lose it," and in fact, Chapter 5 discusses how to draft an incentive plan to encourage managers to save even more.

The reconstituted hiring committee requires clear rules of its own about what it can approve, what it should enforce, and how it should do so. The official productivity policy in Chapter 5 will firmly establish the rules concerning what happens when standards are repeatedly violated absent reasonable grounds. This would be a vast improvement over what is now widely perceived to be an unfair game in which the politically skilled and articulate give "testimony" and get what they want. Once the rules are in place, they are relatively permanent, not easily subject to new policy directions and the *crisis du jour.* The intentional design of some inflexibility in the system will actually maintain and improve performance over time. This gives the organization effective control over its largest item of expense.

The new rules and procedures send a clear and unambiguous message to department management that the ability to make change and the accountability for results rests on their shoulders alone. Financial analysts can advise and assist, vice presidents can offer support, but managers are in charge. The managers will reap the fruits of their success and bear the consequences for coming up short.

Managers will not abuse their authority. They will deliberate greatly before hiring for fear of violating standard. They will wait until they are sure volume is permanently high enough to justify new hires or authorizing more overtime or registry. They will stop the constant requests for more people and find ways to do more with the same staff. An incentive system proposed in Chapter 5 will offer encouragement to run better than standard.

Terms of the Deal

Every department manager is responsible for meeting productivity and cost standards that are 100% variable or 100% fixed. This is an either/or proposition, a manager cannot have both in the same department. Either labor hours are flexible with some volume indicator or they are not. Mixing these two concepts has rendered traditional productivity systems ineffective. This is the simplest and most easily understood staffing system. It is intuitive and fits with how managers run their departments. For variable departments, which normally comprise all of the nursing and ancillary units, standards are simple and clear: labor hours per unit of service and labor cost per unit of service (excluding vacation, sick, holiday, and benefits). For fixed departments, total hours and total labor cost are the standards.

Department managers decide whether fixed or variable would suit their departments best. If the analyst or consultant understands the workings of the department, he or she will be able to advise managers of what will likely work best. If managers opt to be fixed, they get the traditional budget of total labor hours and dollars. Departments that have some easily measurable and workable unit of service would generally be unwise to choose an all-fixed department, because they would be caught short-handed if volume increased beyond budgeted expectations. If managers settle on variable, total labor will flex up and down with volume, multiplied by the hours and cost per unit standards. Few departments may switch from fixed to variable, or the reverse, but it is their choice. Where the manager should have made a different choice, the decision can simply be reversed. This will be rather infrequent, but nothing is carved in stone. Departments will be monitored according to the fixed or variable method they choose.

Department managers can hire on their own authority, but they will be accountable for meeting standards. As discussed previously, authority and responsibility must be equally matched. Funding for new positions or new functions will continue to need committee approval based on the merits of the case.

Implications for Managers

Fixed departments have a relatively easy time of it—the traditional fixed budget, common to most administrative functions, works quite well. For variable departments, the new productivity system can be a two-edged sword: they can fully staff for workload increases, but they have to downsize for workload decreases—and not part of the way, but all the way. No "fixed" component saves them from having to scale down to meet reduced demand. If they get 30 minutes per test and they experience a reduction of 10 tests per day, they will need to reduce staffing by 5 hours per day.

If volume temporarily turns very low, managers, supervisors, and anyone else skilled at patient care will be expected to don a smock, roll up his or her sleeves, and get on the floor, up close and personal with the patients. This is where "fixed" staff becomes variable. There is nothing wrong or humiliating about managers and supervisors occasionally doing other jobs; even those tasks normally done by those lower in rank and status. No one should be above doing whatever is needed to help. That shows real leadership. Clerks and secretaries can even flex up and down to support the department. No longer is the fixed/variable skill mix centrally managed, and the department manager is solely responsible for meeting cost and hours standards. If volume regularly becomes very low, combining departments to make a larger, potentially more efficient unit might be worth a serious look. These are the kind of operational questions that should be asked in the quest for better productivity.

What hour and cost standards should be used? The same figures that were agreed on in the meetings and negotiations with department managers (see Chapter 2). What worked so well as an analytical tool should carry forward into standards development. It would be wise to maintain continuity with the analysis instead of jumping to some other way of developing standards and subsequent monitoring. Translation of figures from one method of calculation to some other is unnecessary and undesirable, and many productivity improvement projects have failed over the long run for this very reason. The integrity of the standards must not be compromised.

Organizations should also pass up the temptation to achieve some arbitrary target by "shaving" the standards to make labor costs fit an organization's objective. Someone may compute that $250,000 more can be saved by subtracting a tenth from each department's standard, for example, by going from 9.6 hours per unit to 9.5. Although very tempting—it looks like easy money—the integrity of the system will be destroyed, along with trust. On a related note, it is best to avoid carrying the figures to three decimal places, as in 9.561 hours per patient day, implying a mathematical precision that does not exist in human affairs. Two decimal places are plenty of precision; one may be even better.

What Is in it for Us?

With new autonomy and freedom come new obligations. To managers unaccustomed to such focused accountability, it may seem a bit intimidating. Either the complexity of the budgeting and productivity system previously let them off the hook, or the approval process shifted the burden of responsibility onto someone else. Now, they have to manage resources rather carefully.

To others, such power and responsibility will come as a liberating and most welcome change. It all depends whether a manager is a bureaucrat or an entrepreneur at heart. Entrepreneurial behavior can be brought out of hiding if people are put in that position. Either way, the job of administrators is to guide and train their managers and support them in this new order so that all can be responsible. Perhaps more important than the financial effect produced is the trust such a move can create with middle managers. They now have some of the authority normally reserved for those more senior. The new power is at once liberating and confining—freedom balanced with consequences. That is exactly what the new organization should want to instill in all of its managers.

The new regime offers solid advantages for managers that should be heavily promoted. These advantages provide balance, offering something to managers in return for accepting individual responsibility. These advantages make the new system more persuasive overall than the alternative of simply doing nothing.

- If department volume increases, managers are automatically entitled to match it with more staff hours. That does not mean they must match it, only that they can. If their standard specifies 30 minutes per test, then ten more patients will merit 5 more hours. No "fixed" component will hold them back (it never really did anyway—they would get permission for additional hiring eventually).

- The skill mix is theirs to manage as they see fit, provided, of course, that cost per unit is managed to standard or better. The contingent of "fixed" staff—manager, clerk, and secretary—is theirs alone to determine.

- They do not have to beg permission to hire, a sore point among middle managers. They are not put in the position of supplicants. As trusted and valued employees, managers will now exercise control with responsibility. They can hire on their own authority, but they must also accept the self-governing restraint that comes along with it, similar to the restraint faced by any business owner.

- Managers should be told that their standards are permanent—unless the organization engages in a formal benchmarking study in which real activities and tasks are changed in order to drive further performance improvement. This is very important, because trust will be established no other way. If managers are able to be beat their standards, and many of them will, then they will operate with a favorable variance. That is a good thing! Yet, organizations reward a manager who comes in under standard with a smaller budget the next year, virtually guaranteeing that a favorable variance will never happen again. Managers should not be encouraged to spend the maximum via perverse incentives. The standard should be considered a ceiling, not a floor.

Many managers will run their departments with a comfortable margin of error, and administration should encourage that. Most managers will exercise authority with responsibility wisely and conservatively; more conservatively, in fact, than in the present system, in which they give "testimony" at the first opportunity. Most managers will rarely come into conflict with their standards, and productivity will cease to be the major headache it has been up until now. With favorable variances encouraged, it might surprise some how managers will find ways to exceed their standards. Allow them to do so!

Management discretion does currently exist; it is just invisible because managers spend up to the limit for fear of losing their budget. By making the standards relatively permanent, fear dissolves, and managers are free to turn out better than standard performance, without any negative consequences. In fact, the incentive system proposed in Chapter 5 encourages, not penalizes, better performance. Once standards stop changing from year to year, and people are truly held accountable, not just in word but in deed, then executives may be surprised at how the rush of new hires slows and virtually ceases as productivity is brought under control. Managers will apply discretion and not recklessly leap into a hiring frenzy. They will start thinking as owners, not employees.

Essentially, the old thinking was this: "If I hire more people, my job and that of my crew becomes easier. It will be less stressful for us. The organization always seems to find the money to spend on other things. My request is just a drop in the bucket. They'll find the money for me too." This is destructive, but all-too-common, thinking. When all managers adopt this attitude, the organization enters a dangerous cost spiral. This is not the company culture that is wanted.

The new thinking goes something like this: "If I hire new people, it might make my job a little easier, but do I have the volume to support it? Do the numbers justify it? Has something fundamental to my business suddenly changed? What if my volume increase is just temporary? I could end up bringing in new people and then go over my standard. Then I would have to let my new people go, which would be unfair. I had better wait a few more weeks to see whether the new patients we are getting are a permanent increase. Maybe we could rearrange our schedules more in line with our patients. That might allow us to exceed our standards comfortably."

The new organizational culture pushes everyone to think like the CEO, making the same decisions a CEO would make, reacting to the same incentives and consequences as a CEO. If the organization can get its managers to think like this, then it will have conquered its productivity problems.

Rules for Changing Standards

Labor standards provide ample protection against undesirable, costly change. Standards, however, should not be set in stone. At some point, new business conditions or profitable opportunities will arise, and the organization needs some flexibility to capitalize on them without rigid standards preventing welcome change. The organization may, for example, add new programs, functions, or services to existing departments, or it may choose to improve the level of service currently provided.

One of the former hiring committee's new roles is authorizing changes to department standards, but it needs clear procedures to avoid recreating the testimonial process. These procedures provide guidance to help distinguish actions that would violate a manager's existing standard from those that would not. The committee would weigh approval according to measurable cost–benefit criteria. Here are the questions executives and managers alike would ask when deciding if a department's standards should be changed.

- *Will a new hire violate the standard?* If not, the manager is free to hire without approval. Whether vacancies or increased patients create a favorable variance to standard is no longer an issue. If a new hire can be accommodated within the current standard, there is no need to revise the standard.

- *Has volume increased (variable departments)?* If so, the manager can staff for it as the standard allows. With more volume, the existing standard will accommodate more hours, and the manager does not need permission to hire. He or she should take care not to staff beyond what volume allows. In this case, no adjustment to standard is needed.

- *Is this a new, non–volume-related position?* Managers may want to hire people for new functions that have no direct connection to workload volume. A manager may, for example, want to hire a quality control specialist, or the finance department might want another analyst. If the department has been running a favorable variance, there may be room for such new hires, and the standard does not need to be changed. If not, then new hires for non–volume-related functions will violate the standard, and the manager needs to make a good case for an increase to his or her standard. In these situations, the executive review committee should employ some type of cost–benefit analysis to ensure that the organization will profit from the investment or that the position will pay for itself—if not in cash, then in some other measurable outcome that executives think is worth the cost. The committee should decide on the exact format of this analysis in advance to avoid becoming embroiled in more testimonials. The idea is to employ the same logic as in a small business, in which the cost impact would be obvious and immediate.

It is best to look on these new personnel costs as an experiment. Measurable financial or quality improvement goals ought to be agreed on and regularly monitored. The committee should follow up after 6–12 months and see how it is working to ensure the organization is getting a return on its investment. If so, the experiment would be deemed a success. If it turns out not to be worthwhile, the experiment should be terminated by deploying the new people elsewhere, or by letting attrition solve things over time, so that the department is brought back into balance. How often is this done now? It is much more likely, having made the decision to hire, that the whole episode is forgotten and never revisited. This establishes a bad path for others to follow—promise a lot, but do follow up.

Getting managers to think about measurable targets may give them pause, but it is very worthwhile for everyone to know exactly what it is that they are committing themselves to achieve. Is it not reasonable to ask that the justification for new hiring prove itself?

Many managers will pose the question: Can we hire now for planned volume? This is reasonable for new programs, in which there is often a minimum staffing level needed while the program works up to a steady patient load. Advance recruiting is usually necessary. Perhaps service volume will expand with the addition of a new doctor on staff. People may need to be brought on board and trained before the patients start arriving. Over time, as volume builds, productivity will be fine, but until then, there will be more staff than needed for the actual patient load. What ought to be done?

The solution is simple: treat the department as fixed for the time being or grant a temporary waiver. Some departments and functions should be exempt from the productivity system (the fourth performance category in Communicating the Findings, Chapter 2). Productivity reports will still be produced for them, but they will be treated differently than the rest. New programs should have a business plan that lays out the hiring schedule that can be used as a guide for monitoring purposes. When it is necessary to hire in advance of actual need, a waiver can be granted for the time that it takes to realize the volume. Suppose, for example, a manager wants to hire a nurse today for patient volume arriving in 2 months. The solution is to grant a waiver of one FTE for 2 months; in other words, allow a variance of one FTE for 2 months. If the patients should fail to materialize, or come more slowly than expected, the department should reduce accordingly. If the patients do in fact come, then the current standard would suffice. In either case, the waiver is temporary, not permanent, because the position in question, like current positions, is tied to volume.

Sometimes the opportunity arises to hire a person now for a coming vacancy that will be very difficult to fill. The manager has to make a decision, even though the vacancy will not occur for 2 months. Again, a waiver of one FTE for 2 months will take care of the situation. That takes care of temporary adjustments without agreeing to permanent staffing increases. Say, for example, the addition of a new non–volume-related person is intended to maintain better cost control over the department and therefore the position will pay for itself. This may be a new supervisor on the night shift to address lax staffing control. If so, the position can be accommodated within the existing standard within 1 or 2 months, and no permanent change to standard is necessary.

The only conditions that require a change to an existing department standard is the addition of new non–volume-related functions, new programs, or hiring in preparation for future patient volume. For these few exceptions, approval should still be sought so that those managers do not conflict with their standards. Unlike the old testimonial process, managers are required to realize objective and measurable goals as a condition of approval. Although not an impossible hurdle, approval will certainly prove more difficult to obtain than before. For purposes of keeping the lid on labor growth, that is all very well.

The New Deal: Harsh or Kind?

Management systems operate on an implicit worst-case basis. Because *some* managers are not willing to be responsible, *no one* can be responsible. Because *some* managers might abuse their hiring authority, *no* managers may have hiring authority. Because *some* managers might exceed reasonable spending limits, *everyone* must be tightly restricted. Because *some* managers may blunder, *no one* can be trusted. Traditional management philosophies and practices are designed around this fear. Once the organization realizes its control systems are not producing what it wants, it is apt to respond with even more central control, making everything worse.

"WHAT MESSAGE DOES THE PUBLIC GET WHEN THE HOSPITAL IS IN FINANCIAL PERIL? WHILE THE MARKETING PEOPLE WORK TO SHOW OTHERWISE, IS THE HOSPITAL NOT TELLING THE COMMUNITY THAT SERVICE AND QUALITY MAY BE CUT?"

By comparison, the new system offered here is fairer and more equitable than what many organizations have now. It may be tempting to compare the management approach in this book with some ideal alternative that avoids the unpleasantness of assigning responsibility and enforcing compliance. It will never happen. There is no viable alternative. Productivity problems will not go away. They must be tackled successfully for the long-term viability of the organization. Things cannot run themselves; duties and obligations cannot be dodged without chaos arising. Running the organization on an *ad hoc* basis is neither fair to managers and staff, nor is it economically sound. The new system is surely fairer than the inevitable alternative to be faced down the road—layoffs and cuts.

The new management roles are not as scary as they might sound at first. Adults expect control over their personal lives, accepting the responsibility that comes with it—why not in their business lives too? In a matter of months, managers will quickly assume the responsibility and learn to adapt to the new system with its incentives and consequences (proposed in Chapter 5). Via the new monitoring report illustrated in Chapter 4, the organization will have all the control it needs, not by managing the process, but by controlling the outcome.

Which is better—the "kinder" *ad hoc* system, breaching budget discipline, unexpected layoffs and cuts, people waiting on edge for the next inevitable crisis, or a system where managers exercise discretion, control, and responsibility behind the scenes? Which is superior—an institution where things run very smoothly or one where disruption is the order of the day? Would it be better for organizations to stick with the present system in which those who increase their budgets every year eventually provoke a financial crisis that requires drastic action from everyone, even from those not responsible? Or, conversely, would the alternative actually be kinder—a structure of rules, procedures, and standards in which only the most incompetent managers are weeded out. Accountability works if administration is willing to let it operate, mustering the courage to see it through to completion. Old bureaucratic procedures that sufficed in an earlier time must be abandoned as incompatible and expensive in today's cost-conscious environment.

> "THE TIME TO REPAIR THE ROOF IS WHEN THE SUN IS SHINING."
> —JOHN F. KENNEDY

Meeting labor standards should not be an option. Managers can do it because they did it before. It is hard to argue with reality—

after all, the standards were drafted from history, not projections, corporate objectives, or targets.

IMPLEMENTATION STRATEGY

Chapter 1 argued that layoffs have been a failure, a tactic by managements at a loss for what to do. There are viable alternatives that shun layoffs for a smoother transition—one without headlines, strikes, or harmful publicity. The key is recognizing that hardly any financial crisis emerges out of the blue. It only seems that way because the early warning signs are not recognized in time. The existence of a crisis points to the fact that something serious is out of control and has reached the point where it can no longer be ignored. Payer mix changes, shifts in clinical service mix, and other variables can hide the impact of declining productivity. Proper monitoring and ongoing analysis is therefore critical (see Chapter 4). If financial problems take time to evolve, it seems reasonable that solutions should be allowed the time to succeed.

Some administrators want to be seen taking decisive action by making radical changes that will favorably affect next months' financial statements. One of the problems with this is that drastic changes usually prove to be temporary. If the conditions that gave rise to the crisis are not addressed, the problem is bound to recur. It is wiser to pursue a course of action that will result in enduring superior productivity, not a temporary fix.

Relate Productivity to Strategic Goals

Nearly every organization has a *mission statement,* an expression of its core values. These mission statements usually express the organization's commitment to efficiency and effectiveness, its promise to care for all patients regardless of their ability to pay, and a pledge to provide the best-trained staff and technology to the public. These values and principles are further elaborated and quantified in a strategic plan, which includes tactics that spell out how the organization mission will be promoted over the next several years. New services, expansion of existing services, new technology, outreach programs, and the like are featured in the strategic plan.

One of the pillars of any strategic plan is financial strength, without which the organization cannot accomplish any of its other objectives. Financial strength is often expressed as a measurable goal to be achieved within the time frame of the strategic plan. All of management would have been involved in the preparation of the strategic plan and therefore would be intimately familiar with its goals. Furthermore, the board would have signed off on the specific strategic and financial targets contained in the plan. This offers a ripe opportunity to link important strategic and financial goals to productivity.

A major initiative such as the push for superior productivity should not be pursued in isolation. The CEO should make an explicit link between productivity and agreed-on strategic goals, driving home the necessity of improving the organization's cost structure to the attainment of everything else. Because management and the board would have already agreed to increase the organization's financial strength, productivity should be positioned as a central tactic for achieving the organization's critical strategic and financial goals. Now is the time to tie productivity to the organization's mission and strategy. Doing so will help ensure that momentum and urgency are maintained.

Allow for a Transition Period

Recall from Chapter 2 that it takes about 3 months to do a proper analysis, meet with managers, present the results, make recommendations to the executive team, and reach agreement on coordinating implementation. Executives also have to discuss the particulars of the productivity policies for their organizations, then draft and send them out for review, comment, and revision. If all of this were to take place immediately, panic would ensue. Managers might have to trim down quickly by cutting employee schedules or having a quick layoff. Neither of these is recommended. It is smarter to allow for a transition period so that managers can adjust to the new regime and make their plans accordingly in a calm and orderly atmosphere.

In addition, the section titled Communicating the Findings in Chapter 2 demonstrated that only one quarter to one third of all departments will likely be in the Losing Ground group. These form the group of managers who will need to draft new staffing schedules in order to meet standard. Up to 75% of all department managers are relatively unaffected and need make no change, or relatively minor change, to meet standard. They will have to watch productivity carefully and be accountable for maintaining performance, but the whole organization will not go through a sweeping transformation. Only those who need to make some changes are affected.

An informal transition to the new productivity program should have occurred during the analysis phase that lasted about three months. During this time, it should have been apparent to all managers, or at least to the executive hiring committee, that this would be a poor time to staff up. It would be much better to see the results of the analysis, even if preliminary, to know where a particular department stands before submitting a request for new hires. Once standards have been formally enacted, monitoring is in place, and a productivity policy has been adopted, a formal transition period should commence. This "grace" period gives managers the time to make any necessary changes without being penalized from day one. After the transition period, enforcement begins. That said, monitoring against standard does indeed begin on day one. Only enforcement is put on hold.

How Long Should the Transition Take?

A decent transition period is about three months. Any longer and the sense of urgency and momentum is lost. It hints to managers that commitment amongst the executive team is uneven. A deadline way into the future is not much of a deadline. Managers will put off acting until their time is short. Any shorter than 3 months, however, is probably too quick. The goal is to have managers in full compliance with their standards, or nearly so, by the time the grace period ends. They will have a reasonable period during the transition "interlude" to get things in order. A reasonable interval is an indication of thoughtful order and systematic process. It is considerate, and that goes a long way to generating good will.

How long each organization takes in its transition period is, of course, a unique matter. The interval will be specific to the conditions and culture of each institution. The urgency depends on the financial condition of the health care organization and perceptions on the board. A health care organization needing an emergency cash infusion in a desperate turnaround situation will not have the luxury of time that might otherwise exist. This, however, is not the norm. In most cases, it is far more important that the program be launched successfully than it is to save a month or two's worth of excess labor costs. If that consideration or others causes some delay, then so be it. The critical thing is long-term performance to standard, and, with the help of an incentive program to propel change, improving standards over time.

The transition period helps to ensure a smoother landing and optimal longevity for positive results. If the transition period is correct, the organization avoids the costs of severance, outplacement, extended benefits, and so forth that would ensue without a transition period. This also practically eliminates the unquantifiable, but considerable, costs of lowered morale and unscheduled absences that occur when organizations go through troubled times. Paradoxically, then, it may be cheaper to act slowly than quickly. The recommended monitoring interval emphasizes long-term performance by switching to formal quarterly executive evaluations (see Timing of Reviews in Chapter 4). A transition period reinforces the special role that time plays in the productivity management program.

Factor in the Composition of Labor

The composition of labor in each department also affords an opportunity to reach a solution that emphasizes orderly change. In particular, overtime and registry should be analyzed separately to derive a utilization rate, and in terms of overall departmental productivity

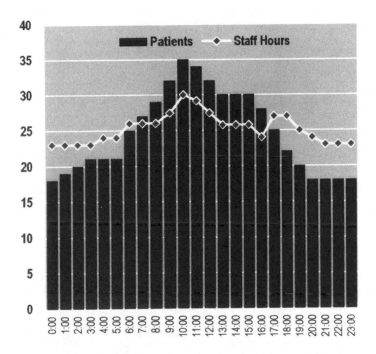

Figure 3.1. Workload distribution analysis. Notice the mismatch of staff and patient load in early morning and late evening hours.

and cost. When savings are indicated, overtime and registry ought to be the first to go. As examined in Chapter 1, one of the most cost-effective ways to cut back on labor expense is to reduce the reliance on overtime and temporary (agency) labor. The organization can save a lot of money by hiring new employees to replace the more expensive overtime, temporary, registry, and perhaps on-call staff. Not only is this approach economically potent, it is relatively painless. Registry employees are, after all, only extra, temporary hands. Overtime use is understood to be occasional, and cutting back saves a lot of money without layoffs or newspaper headlines.

Old rules may have prevented adding new hires, so managers may have found another (more expensive) way to circumvent the rules. With the new rules, sanity can return. The organization should have been tracking overtime and registry labor long ago. If it has not, now is an excellent time to start. As of 2003, reliance on nursing agency labor is at an all-time high. An effective productivity management system will cut into this cost first. These workers are paid up to twice what straight-time workers receive, so a department that can replace an equal amount of premium time with straight time saves a lot of money while leaving total hours unchanged. Many departments can do much better than that, say, by replacing two FTEs of registry with one FTE new hire. If a department has temporary or overtime employees to the extent of one or more FTE, it is time to look at hiring a regular employee instead (see Chapter 1).

The organization should also be aware of the true cost of on-call workers. Because of paid minimums, an on-call employee can be paid three hours to do a half-hour procedure. If this is an occasional instance, then that arrangement is defensible. If, however, a department uses on-call regularly, and at predictable times, then it would be much better to hire a regular employee for the shift, even if a premium has to be paid, and even if the worker is not busy 100% of the time. With the help of an analyst, managers should do the math and decide what is best.

Sometimes, a manager can identify where staffing does not correspond well with patient load. A good tool to identify this condition is the Workload Distribution Analysis (see Figure 3.1). This analysis graphically shows the distribution of labor hours with workload at each hour of the day to identify excess staffing. If there is not a staffing or scheduling system by which to generate the work distribution analysis, such a chart can be assembled with a few months of data gathered from department logs and timesheets. The transition period allows for these kinds of positive activities to occur.

SUMMARY

Although there are legitimate theoretical arguments for splitting staff into fixed and variable categories, they do not hold in real-world practice. Service businesses are not the same as manufacturing, and so-called "economies of scale" are difficult to come by in the health care organization. Commitment and compliance are ultimately more vital than mathematical precision.

Health care organizations should stop taking "testimony," in which a manager pleads for more staff to a hiring committee. An emotional plea is difficult to resist, making it easy to succumb to increased labor costs. With enough patience and shrewdness, managers get what they want in the end anyway. The testimony committee becomes a rubber stamp that promotes labor inflation. More financially sound is reviving the testimony committee to maintain compliance with labor standards. This will be less chaotic and time consuming than current procedures.

In the new system, every department manager is responsible for meeting productivity and cost standards that are 100% variable with volume or 100% fixed. The department manager should make the call. For fixed departments, the standard is total hours and total cost for the year—the normal budget. For variable departments, standards are hours and cost per unit of service. Organizations should avoid the temptation to overengineer it further than this.

Productivity management is not about hardware or software technology, flash reports, or detailed budgets; it is about management. No amount of budget policing can compensate for individual responsibility and accountability. Managers must have the ability to hire on their own authority, but they also must accept ultimate responsibility for their department's performance. Anything less will produce convenient excuses and destroy accountability. Organizations should not worry about a hiring spree; they will retain control through careful monitoring and enforcing compliance to standards. Executives will monitor outcome, not process. Ultimately, the "new deal," with its greater autonomy, accountability, and focus on outcome is fairer and more effective for both managers and executives than a system that relies on top-down, centralized control.

Under certain circumstances, standards should be revised with clear guidelines that help ensure the organization is getting its money's worth. The creation of objective goals followed up by monitoring make certain that they are achieved.

If financial problems take time to evolve, it seems reasonable that solutions should be allowed the time to succeed. A quick fix will not result in enduring superior productivity. A transition period allows managers to adjust and plan accordingly. An informal transition should have occurred during the analysis and meetings phase that lasted about three months. Once standards have been formally enacted, monitoring is in place, and a productivity policy has been adopted, a formal transition period should commence. This second transition phase should take about three months as well. If the transition period is correct, the organization avoids the costs of severance, outplacement, and extended benefits. After the transition period, enforcement begins.

When savings are indicated, overtime and registry ought to be the first to go. Not only is this approach economically potent, it is relatively painless. The organization should have been tracking overtime and registry labor long ago. If it has not, now is an excellent time to start.

MONITORING AND REPORTING

Acceptance of a complex productivity system will always be wanting. The arcane language of management engineering is largely impenetrable to department managers, the very people charged with using the system. People simply will not support what they do not understand. Complex productivity systems, though perhaps intriguing and mesmerizing, are riddled with unintended consequences. The productivity system ought to be simplified so that understanding and commitment are realized; these must be the principal goals.

It takes a great deal of energy to maintain a conventional productivity monitoring system. It becomes corrupted and needs to be overhauled regularly. In contrast, the new monitoring system presented in this chapter is straightforward and built to last. Reports should not be so complex that managers and executives need an industrial engineering degree!

SEDUCED BY TECHNOLOGY

Commercially available productivity systems can measure and report in immense detail, even on the hour. Some are quite sophisticated, even ingenious in their detail and complexity. All of them strive to treat labor measurement and monitoring as a precise science. The premise is seductive to those with a mechanical bent: program, control, and monitor. They have a certain intuitive appeal that keeps customers buying. These information systems would seem to solve some basic problems very conveniently, and they use computerized interfaces and other sophisticated technology!

Conceivably, such systems could help introduce needed discipline and eliminate arbitrary judgment with "machine wisdom." Maybe the real issue, however, revolves around not setting clear objectives for managers, compounded by giving them little authority to follow through. Whom should the organization put in charge—the managers or the software?

TECHNOLOGY AND GOOD MANAGEMENT

It is worth considering exactly what health care organizations hope to achieve with the use of technology. Although sexy, technology cannot replace common sense, whose enemy is needless complexity. Modern technology can deliver complexity by the bushel. While technology can be usefully employed to automate drudgery, it is not particularly useful for advancing knowledge and wisdom. The programmed approach of productivity systems works well for machines, but the actual behavior of human beings working in a service industry like health care is difficult, even impossible, to model precisely. The precision implied by such systems, which may measure hours per unit to the thousandth decimal place, is an illusion.

The principal prerequisite for successful productivity management is not computers, reports, or data. Rather, people must have the authority to act and to learn from the consequences of their decisions. The real question of effective learning is not so much of speed but of motivation, skill, and developing good judgment. Motivation is enhanced when people are accountable for results; skill comes with experience, and judgment is the result of much experience. This has nothing much to do with reams of data, reports, or instant on-demand information. Technology can supply essential data and information, but it cannot make people smarter or wiser. When it comes to productivity monitoring, the organization is well advised to keep the technology as simple as possible in favor of devoting its resources toward developing old-fashioned wisdom, maturity, and skill in all areas. The siren call of fancy graphics and charts are no substitute. Organizations seem to have misplaced a lot of their trust in software. They would be much better off forming their own solutions and fitting them into their own management principles, operating procedures, and official policies so that every manager understands the rules the organization has chosen to guide its actions.

> "THE COMPUTER IS A MORON."
>
> —PETER DRUCHER

Careful attention should be paid to the underlying management philosophy of such systems because what is measured, and how often, carries with it an inherent management method. If the emphasis is on exacting, precise measurements available real-time, on the hour, the organization will be led to adopt intense top-down micromanagement as its business model. This would de-emphasize individual accountability in favor of centralized control, leaving the organization highly unlikely to yield the results it is pursuing. If, however, the monitoring system is simple and understandable, acceptance and accountability will be enhanced. Greater management accountability will mean better management results.

COMPLEX SYSTEMS DO NOT WORK

Although billed as a tool for department managers, complex productivity monitoring systems actually function as a "report card"

> "IT IS A SIMPLE TASK TO MAKE THINGS COMPLEX, BUT A COMPLEX TASK TO MAKE THEM SIMPLE."
>
> —MEYER'S LAW

for oversight purposes. Even as a report card, however, there are severe limitations for managers and executives alike: The more complex and detailed the system, the more confusion. The organization cannot increase accountability unless its managers accept the monitoring system, understanding exactly what it is that they will be accountable for. In an effort to increase accountability, many organizations mistakenly opt for frequent, very detailed reports. What they end up doing is enhancing centralized control, which proves to be self-defeating.

Overengineered productivity standards are unworkable in practice, and minute, detailed monitoring harms, rather than helps, accountability. What is needed is not a better report card, but a simplified, realistic system that managers can understand and accept. When this is achieved, executives will be in a far better position to monitor the results and ensure superior outcomes.

The Law of Unintended Consequences

Most commercial systems now on the market cost upwards of $500,000 for a medium-sized hospital, not including the staff and management costs of implementation, training, annual licensing, software and hardware updates, troubleshooting, and required maintenance. After spending $500,000 and several years from purchase to full utilization, an organization can install a sophisticated monitoring and reporting system. Having invested a sizeable amount of time, effort, and money, organizations have a right to realize their original intent, which is not merely to install a data system. So what do organizations get for their time and money?

Simply put, they get exactly what they paid for: mathematical perfection. Given assumptions keyed in from the budget department, the new system, for example, could compare the actual usage of a "Tech II" to that which the calculations expect. It could compare the average hourly wages of the "Tech II" job class against that which is budgeted. It could automate the preparation of forecasting accrued vacation time for each employee to make scheduling summer vacations easier. It may help to reduce payroll errors and save time preparing paychecks. All nice things to be sure, but it is a safe bet that customers probably do not purchase big systems for any of these reasons.

"The law of unintended consequences," coined by Nobel prize–winning economist Milton Friedman, states that actions intended to attain a certain outcome often achieve the exact opposite result. Surely, the major reason for technologically sophisticated labor management systems, their very reason for being, is to confer precise control of labor costs. Yet, control is primarily a management issue, not a technical or systems problem. Mathematical perfection is no substitute for management responsibility and accountability, old-fashioned though such notions may be. In this case, paradoxical as it may appear, intense budgeting precision and monitoring leads to a flight from individual responsibility. The more managers are dictated to, the less responsibility they can or will assume and the worse the results. They devote their efforts to defeating the budget police, finding ways around the supposed discipline of the monitoring system. Managers can always blame incorrect assumptions about labor mix, pay rates, and patient volumes, largely the baffling work of the budget department anyway. The promised control ends up defeating itself. That is precisely what is not wanted.

TIMING OF REVIEWS

It can take a while for managers to recognize when volume changes give cause for an adjustment to staffing to match the new workload. When volume is suddenly high, managers cannot react immediately to what might turn out to be a temporary episode of greater activity. Until they can catch up, their departments are more productive. Managers cannot react instantly to slower activity either, and until they adjust staffing to match workload, they are less productive. During slower periods, managers have to decide if the reduced volume is a minor fluctuation or a normal seasonal trend, and they tend to be somewhat less productive as they sort it out. Over time, as managers recognize and then react appropriately to changes in workload, productivity evens out.

In practice, the time lag usually means brief periods of above-average and below-average productivity. These variations are especially pronounced day to day. Were the organization to measure productivity every day, it would see far more volatility than over the course of two weeks, the most common interval (it matches the bi-weekly payroll cycle). Two weeks is still a relatively short time. Over longer intervals, volatility cancels out and an undistorted trend is revealed. The rule is: the shorter the period, the greater the volatility. To avoid spotlighting timing differences and normal staffing and workload fluctuations, the timing of productivity reviews needs serious consideration.

Statistically speaking, the productivity ratios in the new all-variable system are somewhat more volatile than under a traditional system. How much more volatile depends on how much the current system grants as the fixed proportion of a given department. For those with a small amount of time now designated as fixed, say 10%, there is not much difference between the old and the new in terms of volatility. For departments with a high proportion of fixed time now included in the current standard, say more than 30%, the ratios of cost and hours per unit of service will be more volatile in the new system. The fixed portion of the department, absent in the new system, acts as a cushion that evens out the ratios. Since most managers do not really understand the current system of fixed and variable hours and costs anyway, it probably does not matter too much, but it still has to be taken into account. This can be done simply by lengthening the timing of reviews.

All statistics are subject to this volatility/duration rule. The weather, for example, is quite variable day to day, but it is certain that the winter will be colder than the summer. The stock market moves up and down day to day; but the long-term trend over the last 60 years has been upward. Long-term investors use that to their advantage, ignoring fluctuations as meaningless background noise to the bigger picture. In productivity analysis, the same applies. Organizations should break away from the 2-week reporting cycle rut, and adopt longer-term horizons for analysis and action. It is wiser to take the long-term view of things.

Productivity should certainly not be monitored every day. There needs to be a clear distinction between real, underlying trends and management problems from statistical variation and artifact. That is why elaborate systems that track productivity by shift are fundamentally flawed—not in arithmetic, but in concept. The short time spans of such reports merely act to highlight timing differences, unexpected staffing and workload fluctuations, and so forth. Rather than a tool that enables organizations to tighten up, they serve to emphasize all that is out of the manager's control and they supply hard figures to make the case! They shift the focus away from management responsibility and toward the measurement system. That is not wanted. More detail and short evaluation periods are counterproductive.

If 2-week monitoring intervals do not accurately represent how the year will finish, why do it? For purposes of executive oversight, to determine if a department is on course or off track, bi-weekly reports will not suffice. Realistically, a quarter's worth of data is needed to evaluate a real trend or a problem that requires action. Commercial industry reports its performance to the markets quarterly because this allows better quality analysis than bi-weekly or monthly periods would allow. Health care organizations should follow the same scheme. Over the course of a few months, volume swings are not that dramatic, and managers have time to adjust to changed circumstances. Over a fiscal quarter, temporary timing problems and statistical aberrations that obscure reality are eliminated and any extra volatility from an all-variable/all-fixed system compared to conventional bi-weekly measurement systems is rendered insignificant.

The best route is to monitor productivity each quarter in a formal group review amongst senior management, using quarterly rollups of the new monthly reports illustrated later in this chapter. The former hiring approval committee that once took testimony should be used for this purpose instead. In the interests of full disclosure, every department's costs and productivity figures should be shared throughout the organization. Organizations ought to stop treating financial reports as secret documents to be shared only on a need-to-know basis and highlight the successes that individual managers achieve, showing what their contribution means to the organization. Administration should celebrate success, encourage the development of a "star" culture, and let everyone see by example what it means to thrive in the new organization.

Reporting Frequency

Executives accustomed to weekly or even daily productivity reports may be uncomfortable with monthly reporting and quarterly reviews. Some executives may feel that things will get out of control if they personally are not on top of everything, everyday. If they wait "too long," things will get out of hand; chaos will ensue. While these are understandable feelings, the opposite is true. If vice presidents control everything, then everyone has to come to them for a decision. In a perpetuating cycle, things will indeed get out of control if they are not intimately involved in making every decision, which is a practical impossibility. It is recommended that executives ease back on the controls and delegate authority and responsibility instead.

Department managers usually want reports more frequently than quarterly. Monthly productivity reports produced alongside the monthly financials are sufficient to keep on top of things. The majority of managers will be content with monthly frequency. Reports more frequent than monthly can become a nuisance, but for those managers who feel otherwise, reports can be tailored to their individual needs. Many managers keep logs of staff schedules and patients, and the financial planning or budgeting department can help put their figures in a format that ties into the productivity monitoring system for tracking productivity using any period desired. Administration should be eager to offer managers any kind of report, of any frequency that they desire. This will help eliminate all excuses for poor performance. If once-a-month reports are one of those excuses, this can be remedied easily enough.

Reports more frequent than monthly should be the department manager's *private tools*. It is not appropriate for senior managers to review bi-weekly productivity reports. If senior managers get involved in the department manager's business, they effectively remove responsibility from the department manager and place it on themselves, which is not desirable from either a practical or a management point of view.

THE NEW PRODUCTIVITY REPORT

One of the problems plaguing productivity improvement programs is tracking progress toward goals. All too often, great effort and time are spent trying to work out a standard of performance for each department, which is then promptly defeated in the monitoring. Often a standard will be worked out using one method of analysis and then translated into completely different units of service for monitoring.

Suppose that a department has all of its various responsibilities sorted into three main groups of tasks and a time value is assigned for each. If it were to stop right there, there would be a standard for each of the three different tasks in the department. If an accurate and timely count of the three tasks could be done, a monitoring report could be developed that would allow the manager to review progress against standard the same way as it was originally developed. A monitoring report that lists each of these tasks would be consistent with the productivity study. This is not, however, what usually happens. More likely, hours worked for each task would be aggregated and translated into hours worked per procedure or other sole workload statistic. This might simplify measurement, but it cuts the link between the productivity study and monitoring. Even though such a translation "works" mathematically, it will hinder acceptance and understanding. This has to be avoided at all costs.

The monitoring report must follow the same format as the original productivity study. If patient days were used to develop the standard, then the monitoring report must reflect patient days. If treatments were the workload unit used, then treatments must remain the yardstick. If not, managers will surely be confused, and a lot of wasted energy will be spent trying to convince them otherwise. Not only that, but also as the link between the productivity analysis and the monitoring report gradually fades over time, no one will be able to justify the standard in use, and the whole project will have to be repeated in a few years.

It is smarter to work backward from the monitoring report when doing the study in the first place. If many different units of measure will not be used in the monitoring, then the productivity study should not measure a host of different things that will not be used. Referring back to the section Assign Performance Measures in Chapter 2, simplicity and continuity of method—from analysis to implementation to monitoring—will get the organization off to a much faster start and greatly aid cooperation.

HOW TO CREATE YOUR OWN REPORT

If the organization does not already have a commercial monitoring system, monitoring reports can be created in-house. The same general ledger accounting systems used to produce cost center reports can be modified to produce an excellent productivity report for every department. Most systems have a "report writer" feature that allows the creation of custom-made reports not available from the vendor. A spreadsheet replica can be created to get the calculations and the basic format right and then transferred to the general ledger's report writer for monthly production. Because it is part of a tested and reliable system already in place, there is little or no maintenance involved once it is set up. Advantages over commercial systems include no licensing fees, multiple-year contracts, high-powered computers, or dedicated analysts required to maintain the system.

The concept of the new reporting is to migrate from two systems and two reports—one productivity report and one cost center financial report—to a single, merged report. The monthly cost center reports provide a convenient vehicle. By using the report writer feature available on most general ledger financial systems, organizations can design their own productivity report, attach it to the back of each cost center summary, and deliver to each manager a single report, eliminating the discrepancy and reconciliation problems attendant with bi-weekly reports. It does away with the misunderstanding caused when the productivity report leads managers to one conclusion and the cost center report leads them in the opposite direction (in which case managers will either pick the most favorable or ignore both). It provides a unified message and reduces unnecessary mailings, distributions, and questions.

If a health care organization wishes to continue using its present productivity system, it can of course do so with fine results. It may be best to make maximum use of what is already in place. The existing system can be optimized in accordance with the principles discussed so far: every department must be either variable or fixed, but not both in the same department. The same reporting frequency should apply if the organization continues to use its present productivity system. The resulting productivity report can look similar, and display the same elements, as the sample report presented in this chapter.

Format of the Productivity Report

The sample report represented in Figure 4.1 connects with the original productivity analysis from Chapter 2. Although simple, it shows everything needed, and eliminates all the superfluous items normally found on such reports. Intuitive simplicity is the whole point. Simplicity aids understanding and therefore compliance.

As illustrated, the new report has two sections: five columns for the current month and five columns for the year to date. Actual performance forms the reference point in the first column, followed

> "FORM FOLLOWS
> FUNCTION."
>
> —LOUIS HENRI SULLIVAN

by budget and standard. The standard takes into account actual volume, not budgeted volume. The rationale is that cost and hours per unit are under management control, but volume is not—at least not at the department level—so an allowance is made for actual volume. Managers have to work with the patient load they actually have, not what the budget projected. The standard represents what the organization would have budgeted with perfect knowledge of actual volumes. Organizations may choose to add some extra columns, such as "percent difference" or "prior year" or others along those lines. It has been simplified here to enhance understanding.

Note the additional step of including benefits, supplies, and other expenses on the same report. This way, total expenses on this part of the report agree with the rest of the cost center report. Benefits and supplies are normally variable with volume, and other expenses are usually fixed, as they are here, but can be divided any way the organization wants to. More detail is usually found on the same cost center report, such as the overtime or registry percentage, holiday pay, and so forth. If not, it may be a good idea to incorporate it into the productivity monitoring report.

By creating its own report, the organization can customize the report to suit its preferences. Whatever will aid understanding should be incorporated. It might be a good idea to ask managers what they would like to see included, just so long as the focus is not lost on hours and cost per unit of service. Decision support systems can charge a tidy sum for purchasing a productivity module like this, but organizations can do it themselves for nothing.

How to Analyze the Report

As shown in Figure 4.1, managers and analysts can underscore productivity and salary problems in moments. Management is immediately aware of the cost of productivity losses (or the amount saved) for each department. These amounts can be summed for the organization each month. What does the sample report show? The department is doing well against budget, but only because budgeted patient volume is higher than actual. As it turned out, the budget gives the department more than it really needs, because volume is lower than projected. Put another way, the department should be handily beating its budget. A simple budget variance figure, unadjusted for the difference between budgeted and actual volume, obscures the reality of the situation.

Against the standard, there are a few problems. Year to date, the department paid out more than 6,000 additional labor hours

Total

	Current Month			Better/(Worse) Than		Year to Date			Better/(Worse) Than	
	Actual	Budget	Standard	Budget	Standard	Actual	Budget	Standard	Budget	Standard
Patient Days[1]	270	283	270	(13)	0	2,768	3,146	2,768	(378)	0
Productive (Worked) Hours[2]	5,805	6,260	5,972	455	167	66,442	69,590	61,237	3,148	(5,205)
Non-Productive Hours	960	1,019	972	59	12	10,813	11,326	9,966	512	(847)
Total Paid Hours	**6,765**	**7,279**	**6,944**	**514**	**179**	**77,255**	**80,915**	**71,203**	**3,660**	**(6,052)**
Productive Salaries[3]	198,450	201,029	191,795	2,579	(6,656)	2,146,064	2,171,841	1,911,165	25,777	(234,899)
Non-Productive Salaries	32,819	31,280	29,843	(1,539)	(2,976)	349,269	347,727	305,991	(1,542)	(43,278)
Total Paid Salaries	**231,269**	**232,309**	**221,638**	**1,040**	**(9,631)**	**2,495,333**	**2,519,568**	**2,217,156**	**24,236**	**(278,176)**
Average Hourly Wage	34.19	31.92	31.92	(2.27)	(2.27)	32.30	31.14	31.14	(1.16)	(1.16)
Benefits	21,722	25,453	24,284	3,732	2,562	243,951	282,951	248,990	39,000	5,038
Supplies	18,374	15,214	14,515	(3,159)	(3,858)	145,618	169,129	148,829	23,511	3,211
Other (Fixed) Expenses[4]	7,914	7,981	7,981	67	67	92,741	93,908	93,908	1,167	1,167
Total Expenses	**279,277**	**280,957**	**268,417**	**1,679**	**(10,860)**	**2,977,643**	**3,065,557**	**2,708,883**	**87,913**	**(268,760)**

(continued)

Per Unit	Current Month			Better/(Worse) Than		Year to Date			Better/(Worse) Than	
	Actual	Budget	Standard	Budget	Standard	Actual	Budget	Standard	Budget	Standard
Productive (Worked) Hours	21.50	22.12	22.12	0.62	0.62	24.00	22.12	22.12	(1.88)	(1.88)
Non-Productive Hours	3.56	3.60	3.60	0.04	0.04	3.91	3.60	3.60	(0.31)	(0.31)
Total Paid Hours	**25.06**	**25.72**	**25.72**	**0.66**	**0.66**	**27.91**	**25.72**	**25.72**	**(2.19)**	**(2.19)**
Productive Salaries	735.00	710.35	710.35	(24.65)	(24.65)	775.20	690.35	690.35	(84.85)	(84.85)
Non-Productive Salaries	121.55	110.53	110.53	(11.02)	(11.02)	126.16	110.53	110.53	(15.63)	(15.63)
Total Paid Salaries	**856.55**	**820.88**	**820.88**	**(35.67)**	**(35.67)**	**901.36**	**800.88**	**800.88**	**(100.48)**	**(100.48)**
Benefits	80.45	89.94	89.94	9.49	9.49	88.12	89.94	89.94	1.82	1.82
Supplies	68.05	53.76	53.76	(14.29)	(14.29)	52.60	53.76	53.76	1.16	1.16
Other (Fixed) Expenses	29.31	28.20	28.20	(1.11)	(1.11)	33.50	29.85	29.85	(3.65)	(3.65)
Total Expenses	**1,034.36**	**992.78**	**992.78**	**(41.58)**	**(41.58)**	**1,075.58**	**974.43**	**974.43**	**(101.15)**	**(101.15)**

[1] Standard patient days equals actual patient days

[2] Standard/actual volume multiplied by budgeted/standard hours per unit of service

[3] Standard/actual volume multiplied by budgeted/standard cost per unit of service

[4] Other expenses are fixed and do not vary with volume; standard and budget are the same

Figure 4.1. New productivity report.

than was justified by its volume; this cost the organization $278,176 more in paid salaries than should have been spent. Year-to-date productive hours were 24.00 per patient day compared with the standard of 22.12. In addition, the year-to-date average hourly wage was almost 4% over standard, $32.30 per hour compared with $31.14 at standard. This may not sound like much, but the wage difference alone adds up to almost $90,000 ($1.16 per hour × 72,255 paid hours = $89,616). Year-to-date hours per patient day and average hourly wages both exceeded standard; the department spent $901.36 in paid salaries per patient day compared to the standard of $800.88. This indicates that in addition to a problem with productivity, there is a problem with skill mix, registry, overtime, or some combination of these. Surely, this is where organizations should focus their attention, instead of getting lost in the details.

MAKE THE MASTER SCHEDULE WORK

The key to maintaining productivity and control of staffing is the master staffing schedule. This schedule prescribes the level of staffing for various patient volumes. Clinical directors should use this schedule as a guideline for staffing depending on the types of patients to be cared for and other considerations. An effective staffing schedule should need relatively few revisions. Managers should be able to follow it almost all of the time. If they do not—or will not—follow it, then there really is no schedule. Without a master schedule, it is more difficult to know if the department is on track.

An effective master staffing schedule does not need to be constantly changed. It anticipates that different days of the week have different workload volumes and staffs accordingly, yet still allows for flexibility as volume and seasons change. On average, following this schedule should consistently produce productivity that is on standard. Automated commercial staff scheduling systems are well worth a look, especially the newer web-enabled kind, but the organization and the department have to make sure beforehand that the software will actually be used. Managers should ask themselves several questions:

- **Does the department have a master schedule?** If not, develop one with clinical and financial staff.

- **How often does the department make exceptions to the staffing schedule?** Some managers make constant changes to their schedules to accommodate their employees' needs. This can, however, easily get out of hand. Rather, the schedule needs to be set up to accommodate the patient's needs. If accommodating employees causes the department to breech its productivity standards, the manager must coax greater flexibility from his or her present employees or prepare to replace them with others who will provide the needed predictability.

- **Is the core-staffing schedule set low to appear extremely productive on paper?** This is an expensive option. Most managers who have tried this have made up the nearly constant shortfall with overtime and registry. The labor standard would already include hours worked for overtime and registry, but likely not at a high, continuous level. Instead, the master schedule should be reset to a more realistic level, so that the department can manage with less overtime or registry. Realistically, employees working long shifts are not as fresh as those starting their shifts, so to the extent that overtime can be replaced with straight time, the department will cost less and be more efficient at the same time. In addition, consider if there is a significant callback component. Even for a procedure that takes a half-hour, the department might be paying for a minimum of three hours. If the manager replaces this three hours with straight time, more staff will be working in the unit at far less cost.

- **Is the master schedule followed by everyone in charge of staffing decisions?** If not, initiate training and guidelines so that all managers and supervisors in the same clinical area are making consistent decisions.

- **Does everyone who sets staffing review the results of their decisions?** It is not enough merely to follow the master schedule; results have to be monitored regularly to know if the department is on track and what changes might be necessary. If results are not being monitored, the manager should develop monitoring tools that would enable those in charge of staffing to learn the consequences of their decisions. Preferably, there would be a regular department management forum, in which managers, supervisors, charge nurses, and others could discuss, learn, and improve from shared experience. No one in a position of leadership should operate in a void.

- **If the department follows the staffing schedule, does it produce the results needed?** If not, the manager should change the staffing schedule so that it consistently produces the productivity the department needs. The manager should meet with his supervisors and financial analyst to design a new schedule that works for the department.

Adjusting Staffing Schedules

As a rule, the staffing schedule should work for the department and its mission, not against it. It should ensure that patients are getting the hours of care they need, but also make certain that the department is properly managing its costs. The manager should have regular productivity meetings established with his supervisors and financial analyst to discern results, patterns, seasonal trends, and new directions that may require an adjustment to the staffing schedule. The smart manager "banks" some hours and dollars when the opportunity arises to balance unexpected work demands later. In the new productivity management system, managers also realize that next year's budget will not be formulated by this year's labor use. Instead, next year's budget will use the same labor standard currently in use. "Use it or lose it" no longer applies, allowing for improved management.

The proper staffing schedule, adhered to with few exceptions, will produce consistent productivity results. Department managers must have complete control to set the staffing schedules that will work for their departments, marshalling the resources under their own initiative to get the job done. It is their responsibility alone.

Guidelines for Fixed Departments

Fixed departments have their staffing set by the fixed annual budget. The process of maintaining staffing in relation to the budget is simpler than in variable departments because there is no volume adjustment and calculation to work out. A fixed department budget has a set number of FTE and labor costs to go with it. Managers should ask themselves several questions to manage their budgets effectively:

- **Are there any problems with overtime or leaves of absence?** One way for a fixed department to exceed its allotment of staff is the unbudgeted addition of overtime or registry (temporary help). If a manager has an absence, and fills it with temporary workers or overtime, he or she needs to watch the number of hours and dollars to avoid going past his or her standard.

- **Are there any vacancies that do not need to be filled right away?** If so, the department will automatically stay within its budget, all other things being equal. Even if there are unfilled positions for a long time, the standard will remain the same for

next year's budget. The manager has no perverse incentives to
rush for a replacement.

- **Is the vacation schedule spread out?** The standard applies to
  productive hours and dollars. The addition of vacation, sick, and
  holiday to produce total paid FTEs is an estimate for the department from past use, and may vary somewhat for the year. Managers should take care when replacing vacation, sick, and holiday absences with overtime or registry if doing so will exceed
  the number of productive hours budgeted for the department.
  Since the department has an extended period with which to
  meet standard, temporary fluctuations in staffing should not
  matter over the long haul.

Labor resources for fixed departments are relatively easy to
manage since staffing does not vary with volume.

SUMMARY

Conventional, detailed productivity reports are poorly understood
and often ignored; the more complex and detailed the system, the
more confusion. Over-engineered productivity standards are unworkable in practice, and minute, detailed monitoring harms,
rather than helps, accountability. Over-engineering shifts the focus
away from management responsibility and toward the measurement
system. The organization cannot increase accountability unless its
managers accept the monitoring system, understanding exactly
what it is that they will be accountable for.

Any effort to enhance centralized control is self-defeating. Instead, organizations need a tool that furthers comprehension. A
monthly productivity report can be created with the report-writer
feature built into most general ledger accounting systems, or the existing monitoring system can be modified to the same end. Expen-

sive commercial systems may deliver mathematical precision, but they cannot confer precise control of labor costs. Control is a management issue, not a technical or systems problem. To be in control, management needs simplicity to aid understanding, combined with accountability for results.

To avoid spotlighting timing differences and normal staffing and workload fluctuations, the timing of productivity reviews needs serious consideration. The rule is the shorter the period, the greater the statistical volatility. Underlying trends that may require management intervention can best be revealed by lengthening the timing of reviews—monthly and quarterly, rather than bi-weekly. Productivity reports should be rolled up each quarter for presentation, discussion, and corrective action by senior management in a formal group review. In the interests of full disclosure, every department's costs and productivity figures should be shared throughout the organization.

Managers who desire more frequent reports than monthly can build reports custom-tailored to their individual needs. These are the department manager's private tools. The financial planning or budgeting department can help put information from patient logs and staff schedules into a format that ties into the productivity monitoring system. Reporting should never be permitted to become an excuse for poor performance.

The monitoring report must parallel the original productivity study from Chapter 2, preserving the connection between the analysis and subsequent monitoring. If many different units of measure will not be used in the monitoring, then the productivity analysis should not measure different things that will not be used afterward. If patient days were used to develop the standard, then the monitoring report must report in patient days. If treatments were the workload unit used, then treatments must remain the yardstick. Simplicity and continuity of method, from analysis to implementation to monitoring, will greatly aid cooperation.

A tool to maintain staffing control is the department master staffing schedule. An effective staffing schedule needs infrequent revisions. It anticipates that different days of the week have different workload volumes and staffs accordingly, yet still allows for flexibility as volume and seasons change. Managers should be able to follow it almost all of the time. Without a master schedule, it is more difficult to know if the department is on track in the intervals between productivity reports.

INCENTIVES
AND CONSEQUENCES

Once productivity standards are implemented and properly monitored, a balanced strategy is needed to encourage superior performance, yet assure adherence to the new system. If managers have no compelling reason to observe their standards, let alone exceed them, they probably will not. Without incentives and consequences in official policy, any productivity program is almost certain to flounder over time. The cost reduction program described in this book involves the kind of change that could be resisted without meaningful incentives. Any system of cost controls, however clever in design, is easily overwhelmed when the organization unintentionally punishes initiative and rewards inaction. These disincentives must be reversed.

Who has primary responsibility? In what manner should they be held accountable? Although managers need clear consequences for poor management, they also need incentives for superior performance. This chapter shows how to establish incentives for superior management and create consequences for poor management. The sample productivity policy in this chapter unites the elements of the book's program. It establishes the ground rules to guide conduct and formally codifies the lines of authority and responsibility at each level of management.

LAYING THE FOUNDATION

Chapter 2 presented the fairest and simplest approach to dealing with productivity. Each department's productivity was analyzed and compared to itself from prior years, what may be called *historical benchmarking*. Every department was declared either variable with workload volume or fixed, not some mix of each. In this way, a map was created of where each department had been and what the impact of changing productivity meant in hours and dollars. All departments were ranked from worst to best. This focused attention on the areas that could improve the most, and the total financial impact was linked to important organizational strategic and financial goals, underscoring the value of developing superior productivity. This logical and clear analytical approach was the basis for a convincing, rational set of practical actions that could be implemented immediately.

Chapter 3 turned to implementation. To what standards, exactly, would managers be held? By implication, the same question was put to division vice presidents. For what, and to whom, were vice presidents to be held accountable? Defining expectations in a clear and unambiguous manner is vitally important. The organization would establish the ultimate accountability of the department manager, who would now have the authority that properly accompanies responsibility. Chapter 3 made the case that department managers should have the autonomy to act while being held accountable to standard. This allows control of the all-important outcome, not the process. The convenient and tired excuses were eliminated to launch a culture of responsibility in the organization, from top to bottom.

For this program to work, administration has to be willing to enforce the rules and not waive them at every chance. It cannot retreat at the first sign of resistance, inviting the old and familiar ways to resume. It was argued that holding managers accountable to an overriding standard renders all other procedures unnecessary and even counterproductive. Defining exactly what the organization wants to achieve in advance, then delegating to and authorizing those responsible for its attainment allows the productivity initiative to succeed.

Now, having framed productivity in terms that allow the organization to solve these interminable problems and having arrived at a practical and workable method, it would be a waste to throw it all away for lack of attention to basic psychology. Without the effect of incentives to motivate people to exceed expectations, or of consequences for not delivering, implementation will fall well short of the potential within reach. The best plan in the world means nothing if the organization is unwilling to demand performance. It does no good to lay down the rules and not follow through. Something extra is needed to cement the new productivity program in place, a system in which managers are actively cooperating, not dragged kicking and screaming.

In most every health care organization, achieving superior productivity—whether defined as meeting historical, internal performance benchmarks or the external benchmarks of industry peers—is a formidable, nearly impossible task. Upon achieving such a goal, however, a new problem emerges: that of maintaining the new level of performance into the future. It is pointless to solve a problem only to have it recur. It is critical to the health care organization's prosperity that it successfully tackles productivity and that, having done so, has a long-term maintenance program.

Maintenance would be a noteworthy improvement over standard practice, but why not raise the bar? If the conventions that held the organization back are demolished, why should it not advance beyond mere maintenance? The goal should be the continual improvement of productivity, year after year. The organization should strive to create the conditions whereby department man-

> "IT IS A FUNNY THING
> ABOUT LIFE. IF YOU
> REFUSE TO ACCEPT
> ANYTHING BUT THE BEST,
> YOU VERY OFTEN GET IT."
> —W. SOMERSET MAUGHAM

agers themselves push for improvement. To get such continual improvement, top-down direction has to be abandoned in favor of a new confidence and trust in the middle managers. Having a comprehensive understanding of their operations, they are ideally positioned to effect positive change. Any disinterest in productivity improvement is entirely due to a lack of incentives. There is no reason to do it. The organization has to get people to stop asking for more, and ask instead how they could do as much, or more, with less.

INCENTIVES

Incentives either work to guide behavior, or they do not. If incentives do work, there should be an incentive plan for every manager so that all are encouraged to work toward the same organizational goals. If, however, incentives are ineffective, then they should be abolished for everyone, including executives. The organization should not be two-faced on the issue. Either everyone can earn incentives, or no one can earn them. This book takes the position that properly designed incentives *do* matter, which is why they are so widely used throughout industry. Incentives encourage the successful achievement of objectives and recognize outstanding contributions to the organization. Lining up incentives throughout the organization allows the setting of priorities that will prove extremely valuable over the long term.

Strictly speaking, people cannot be motivated any more than they can be "learned." They can be taught, but they have to learn on their own and motivate themselves. Administration's job is to create the conditions in which reasonable people would motivate themselves. Action directed toward the achievement of goals is mostly a matter of incentives and disincentives, pursuing positive rewards and avoiding negative consequences. The intensity with which people pursue their objectives is in direct proportion to its real or potential rewards. The opposite of motivation is aimlessness, with neither reward for achievement nor consequences for poor performance.

Most people need some kind of inducement for achieving important goals, whether in business or personal life. In the business setting, rewards encourage the alignment of the individual's goals and that of the organization. What is good for the organization should be beneficial for the individual. Rewards can take the form of bonuses, promotion, respect and admiration, or the inner satisfaction of a job well done. Negative consequences include disapproval, loss of esteem, or economic loss.

Incentives matter! It is human nature to respond powerfully to incentives and consequences. People need rewards for achieving important goals, and they have to face some kind of consequence for poor performance. This keeps people on their toes, striving to improve. The organization ought to structure management jobs to reward the successful and discipline the marginal performers. The alternative is too common: no system of incentives and no consequences—no reward for success, no consequence for mediocrity. This creates a system that kills initiative in favor of inaction, values process over outcome, and drives any entreprencurial spirit out of the organization. Having no incentives or consequences unintentionally punishes the successful and ambitious and rewards those who shun initiative.

End Symbolic Efforts

Insignificant bonuses and suggestion boxes have been used by some organizations in a largely futile attempt to motivate their staff. Devices such as $50 gift certificates or anonymous suggestion boxes to cultivate good ideas are a feeble attempt to overcome something about the organization that powerfully rewards the status quo. Certainly all efforts to extract the best from people, to get them to demonstrate what they can achieve for the organization, should be applauded. Good intentions, however, are not enough. Organizations should end symbolic efforts and put in place genuine incentives that will get the job done.

It would be unwise to count on large numbers of altruistic, exceptionally motivated managers to improve operations. Certainly, it would be nice if all managers were self-motivated to achieve consistent, superb performance, but there simply are not enough of them in any large organization. A plan that rewards able managers while removing under-performing managers would be very desirable. Such a system encourages self-control, not external control. Managers can achieve far more when they direct themselves than when they are ordered. With the right incentives, they will search out and adopt better practices. No program of external, top-down direction can do this nearly as well. The system would integrate individual and organizational goals.

Whatever level of performance the organization is willing to accept will be what it gets. If it rewards superior performance, that is what it will likely get. If it tolerates incompetence, then it will have mediocrity. It is not an issue of good or bad people, or industrious or lazy employees; rather, whatever the organization rewards (or tolerates) will be the order of the day. If superior performance is truly desired, something dramatic has to happen to help pull people in that direction.

> "YOU DON'T START CLIMBING A MOUNTAIN TO GET TO THE MIDDLE. WHY BE CONTENT WITH BEING AVERAGE?"
> —JAMES HART

Why Should We Change?

First, the organization should address the rationale for asking people to change. Why should managers and staff support patient growth and financial objectives? Why should people enthusiastically contribute—not merely attend meetings and sit there, inert, but eagerly collaborate, unite their efforts, and work together? What reason is there to improve? If a compelling reason can be found, then what, exactly, is being improved? How can administration persuade people *not* to hope that its productivity initiative will blow over and die through utter indifference?

The motivational theme that may well be most effective would explain the purpose of profit—not in a dry, abstract sense, but in a meaningful way that relates to people, their motivations, their passions, and their purpose. At nonprofit and investor-owned health care organizations alike, the proposition might run along the following lines:

> We will use the money we save to fund the hospital's mission. We will work to improve patient outcomes. Savings will provide us the means to expand existing services to reach more people and facilitate the development of new medical technologies and life-enhancing services. More funds will enable us to strengthen our community outreach and education and allow us to reward our deserving and dedicated staff appropriately.

Everyone involved in the enterprise benefits, patients as well as employees. All who contribute to the welfare of the organization and its mission, and those who benefit from it, should find the experience enriching. This is not a slogan, but a solemn pledge. Once the savings from productivity improvement are realized, everyone will expect administration to follow through on their pledge by demonstrating how it is using the savings to promote the organization's mission.

Quality Standards

A common objection to incentive plans is that managers will be rewarded for cutting service and quality to save money. Although overblown, it does raise a valid concern. As examined in Chapter 1, severe cost cutting can have a negative effect on medical outcomes. This book takes the position that extreme approaches should be avoided in favor of a more methodical, measured, and sustainable program. Nevertheless, if the organization must overcome unfounded fears that incentives would cause harm, a link should be made between cost and quality, so that one is not obtained at the expense of the other.

Every industry has some generally accepted ways to measure the value that they provide their customers. They do this not because it is the morally correct thing to do, but because they want their customers to come back and to refer to them new customers. They measure and assess their effectiveness to increase the chance of meeting their customer's present and future needs. The profitability of a business depends on its capacity to attract and retain customers. The retail industry, for example, might measure sales returns as one measure of effectiveness. Customers unhappy with some aspect of the transaction reversed the sale. In the manufacturing and production business, the rate of warranty claims might be measured. This tells manufacturers something about their product's reliability and gives them valuable information about the total costs of production (repairs are expensive) and how products might be redesigned to reduce costs and retain customer loyalty.

Health care is not very different from other businesses in this regard. The goal of the organization is obviously not to produce a "cost," even if it is a low cost. Costs can always be cut without regard to its effect on operations or the patronage of doctors and patients. No, the goal of the organization is turning out the best medical outcomes at the lowest cost. How does the organization know that it has successfully attained this goal? If quality cannot be defined and measured, then how is it possible to know if, or even when, managers have achieved their quality goals?

The organization need not carry it too far. If no one is raising the specter of "quality," administration should leave well enough alone. After all, the idea that quality would inevitably suffer with cost standards in place has a fatal logical flaw. If the organization reclaims the cost structure of a given department—historically superior productivity—then quality ought to be the same as it was then. It would not be any worse, especially given the allowance made for any changes to operations (from Chapter 2), and subsequent changes to standards (from Chapter 3). Yet, for managers to argue that quality would suffer, they would have to admit that quality was terrible in the recent past. What manager is going to admit to that? Was overall organization quality appalling just a few years ago? Probably it was not. If the claim were still made that quality would suffer, the manager would have to prove, with before-and- after measurements, that it would be so. He or she cannot simply raise the objection and have administration retreat in fear. There is nothing wrong with presenting valid evidence.

If circumstances dictate that quality is indeed a legitimate concern across a wide swath of the organization, then the organization should consider measurable quality standards for every department to gauge its "mission effectiveness." A compelling measurable outcome would define the services a department performs for its customers, and how well it performs them. This can be paired with cost-reduction efforts so that cost reduction does not hinder the organization's mission.

Outcome does not refer to some bland "statement of values," devoid of any practical on-the-job direction. A statement of a department's outcome should do more than just specify goals for the department. It acts as a means to guide behavior: what, where, how, why, and when. Developing a clear outcome steers employees to achieve their purpose. Without a clear and compelling outcome, employees cannot know why they are doing their jobs. What are they accomplishing? Their job becomes a mere series of tasks to be performed as cheaply as possible. This is an uninspiring and motivationally draining thought.

If the patient accounting manager, for example, were to choose a measure of effectiveness, what might it be? As his or her department's objectives are financial in nature, the measure of mission-effectiveness might be financial as well; perhaps one that relates cost and benefit. The ratio of total cost to total collections might suffice very well, while giving the manager considerable flexibility to achieve the department's goal. This ratio might even become the department's unit of service. The manager could maximize this ratio by reducing cost, increasing collections, or some combination of the two. He or she might even decide to staff up in order to collect even more! This simple ratio would always relate cost with benefit and guide the manager's decisions in the best interests of the organization.

Now consider the perspective of the health care organization president. Costs must be controlled to stay in business. If costs are out of control, where does the president cut? Will there be revenue losses if cuts occur in the wrong place? Will turnaround times extend, delaying discharge and costing the organization more than it saves? Will cuts result in service delays, prompting physicians to move their patients elsewhere? Will the organization's basic mission be impaired? How will the president know the answers to any of these questions without quality measures?

Perhaps the most effective method is to have each manager outline the mission of his or her department, asking each to identify the essential reason that his or her department exists. Alternatively, to ask the question in the negative: What harm would befall the organization if the department ceased to exist? Once the critical mission of the department is identified, the effectiveness of its achievements can be measured as well. It is easy enough to *claim* a given department is critical to the organization and that its mission is being accomplished superbly. It is another thing to *prove* it with objective measurements.

Once there is a consensus within the department on its mission, it should be publicized to reduce the chance of conflicting missions with others. This is the time for coordination and gaining acceptance. Making public progress toward goals also keeps managers on track because a public commitment creates a strong obligation to follow through.

How to Draft an Effective Incentive Plan

With cost and (perhaps) quality standards established, the organization can now turn its attention to systems of reward and risk. An effective incentive plan motivates managers to *exceed* their targets spurs them to accomplish even more. It should automatically reward creativity and innovation. Labor standards only define the *minimum* level of performance an organization will accept. In other words, the organization can quite reasonably insist that performance not deteriorate. Any manager worth keeping, however, can almost certainly surpass the minimum. How far managers can surpass standard is difficult to say, because those not working every day in their departments operate from a position of more limited knowledge.

Many department managers have great ideas for improving productivity, but various obstructions thwart their ideas from becoming reality. Such obstructions include arbitrary budget limita-

---

Current Incentives
- If manager successfully reduces cost, his budget is cut.
- If manager is unsuccessful, he could be fired.

---

tions, capital-spending restraints, and other administrative hurdles. The greatest hurdle, however, is the lack of any incentive to risk making a change, to put forth the effort entailed with improvement. Realistically, managers need some incentive in exchange for the effort.

Consider the management incentives the typical department manager confronts. On the one hand, if he or she successfully reduces cost, his or her budget will surely be cut the next year. The initiative the department manager takes on him- or herself, and his or her success, will be largely invisible. There will be no reward. On the other hand, suppose he or she is not successful, and the cost-reduction efforts are met with apathy or hostility. In taking the initiative to do something in the best interests of the organization, he or she could actually be fired. Why take the risk? The incentive structure is upside down.

An intelligent system of incentives and consequences has three essential components:

1. Highly variable management compensation, with large "upside" potentials
2. Recognition and reward for outstanding performance
3. Departure of the incompetent

Executive Incentives

An executive's main task is to improve the long-term financial and operational performance of the whole organization. Typically, executives are rewarded by annual bonuses, but a more effective incentive plan would be based on a multiyear period to reward long-term, not short-term, performance. This section illustrates such an incentive plan for executives based on achieving the organization's mission.

In the "good old days," CEOs and their executive teams were more caretakers or administrators than entrepreneurs. The primary task was ensuring that daily operations ran smoothly. Organizations were modestly profitable every year, and they were stable places in which to work for a long time. Although salaries may have been

> "INVESTOR-OWNED
> CHAINS, WHOSE
> OPERATING MARGINS
> OUTPERFORM NON-
> PROFITS, RELY HEAVILY ON
> VARIABLE INCENTIVES FOR
> EXECUTIVES."

somewhat less than comparable jobs in industry, without stock options or profit sharing, the security of working for a large, stable organization with regular hours had its attractions. Organizations did not have to worry much about competition, they had a secure slice of the local economy, and as long as people got sick or injured, they were in business.

It is not exactly like that anymore, is it? Yesterday's tranquil cruise is today's wild ride. Many organizations today are not very stable, nor do they offer regular hours. Competitors extend their reach into each other's backyards, doctors are not blindly loyal to the institution, and patients are quite willing to seek alternatives. Medical advances are pushing people to the outpatient setting—quicker, cheaper, and safer—good for patients, but probably bad for business. Cost plus reimbursement is no more. Health care organizations may be full but unprofitable. Security and stability have vanished. With all the tumult, realignments, and restructuring, health care organizations parallel modern industrial corporations. Welcome to the new competitive environment!

Investor-owned health care organizations, meanwhile, are attracting executive talent and paying handsomely for it. Investor organizations pay their executive staff more comparably to general industry; bonus potentials for CEOs may run from 35% to 50%, and the base pay for CEOs is greater at for-profits. This must be having some effect. The for-profit chains, expanding through the purchase of community nonprofit hospitals, may be putting the nonprofit industry at a long-term competitive disadvantage, unless nonprofits are equally prepared to attract and retain first-rate executives.

Relatively few nonprofits offer any long-term incentives for superlative organization performance. In contrast, the rule in industry is to offer a large equity stake with substantial upside potential.

To spur executives to improve the performance of the whole organization, it surely helps if there is an incentive for them to do so. The chief task is to create an ownership ethic where none exists. The ori-

> Based on operating margin percentage, every fifth year executives can earn a percentage bonus applied to their base salary at that time, equivalent to four times the increment in the operating margin percentage of 5 years before.

entation of an owner—the commitment to long-term performance, to brisk growth, and to profit—is a natural outcome of having a stake in the business. In contrast, with nothing at risk and no "upside" potential, hourly wages alone tend to foster security seeking, conservatism, and a reluctance to act. Organizations can change this situation by framing an incentive plan around a desired long-term objective.

Here is an appropriate incentive for executives, based on a target that is easily measurable and of great importance to advancing the organization's mission:

How would this work in practice? If the organization achieved a 5% net operating margin in five years, compared with 2% today, for example, the bonus would be 12% ($5 - 2 \times 4 = 12\%$). If operating margins were 10%, the value of the incentive would escalate quickly to 32%, as illustrated in Figure 5.1 That is a more generous bonus than most organizations might pay today, but the value to the organization is worth many times more than what it cost. It is clearly linked to an easily measurable and objective standard of performance. Moreover, it is flexible. It does not specify what the result *should* be—no specific, arbitrary target is defined. Indeed, specifying an exact target would be limiting because people always have the potential to do better than what they think is possible at the moment. Better to have the incentive open-ended so that executives are encouraged to experiment, learn, and innovate. The incentive re-

		Dollars in Thousands			
		Today	**Hospital in 5 Years**		
Income Statement	Net Operating Revenue	125,000	138,010	144,909	152,082
	Operating Expense	122,500	131,110	134,041	136,873
	Net Operating Income	2,500	6,901	10,868	15,208
	Operating Margin	2.0%	5.0%	7.5%	10.0%
Incentive Package	Total Executive Salaries	1,000	1,159	1,159	1,159
	Percentage Bonus	NA	12.0%	22.0%	32.0%
	Cost of Bonus	NA	139	255	371
	Net Value to Hospital	NA	4,140	7,970	12,167
	Return on Bonus	**NA**	**30:1**	**31:1**	**33:1**

Figure 5.1.   Illustration of an executive incentive plan.

wards improvement. It says that wherever the organization is today, the potential exists to do better.

Net operating margin is a more comprehensive measure of financial performance than revenue growth or expense reduction. It is a combination of the two, within the sphere of executive influence. The incentive is proportional to existing salaries and the value to the organization, producing over thirty times as much as paid in incentives. If the organization fails to improve its operating position, it would pay nothing to the executives in incentives. It pays only for results, so there is nothing to lose.

Figure 5.1 can serve as a template for an organization to design its own incentive plan for executives to replace or modify the one it currently uses. Of course, there is nothing magic about the four times payment formula. It could be more or less, but the idea here is to make the incentive meaningful to the individual and the attainment of the goal important to the organization.

More important than the money is the alignment of interests at all management levels and the setting of priorities that incentives help accomplish. It is not the money so much as what it represents— the successful attainment of important objectives, and recognition for contribution to the organization in proportion to the benefit.

How to do the Calculations:

Percentage Bonus: operating margin in year five minus today's operating margin times four.

Cost of Bonus: percentage bonus multiplied by total executive salaries.

Net Value to Hospital: operating margin in year five minus today's operating margin, times net operating revenue in year five.

Return on Bonus: Net value to hospital divided by cost of bonus.

Manager Incentives

Knowledge and ability are not limited to the executive suite, yet the most widely used incentive and bonus plans reward just the executives, creating the potential for misaligning their interests with that of their managers. Suitable incentives for managers can tap their valuable operating knowledge to improve the organization's performance. This section presents a plan for department managers based on measurable performance improvement.

It is curious that the rationale for executive incentives is the same reasoning used to discourage similar incentives for department managers. If incentives help motivate senior managers to further the organization's goals, why should it not work equally well for those more junior to them? Indeed, why should it not work even better? Department managers have the most direct control over business

"IT IS NOT THE MONEY THAT MATTERS MOST, BUT THE ALIGNMENT OF INTERESTS AND THE SETTING OF PRIORITIES URGENT TO THE HOSPITAL THAT COUNT."

processes, work methods, and procedures, so it makes sense that they would have the most direct control over costs as well. Taking the position that only executives should earn incentives implies that everyone else is negligent or incompetent. Somehow, department managers do not have it in them to respond to incentives. This would be the reason that executives could respond to incentives, but no one else could. Does that make sense?

For the purposes of this chapter, the real difference between middle managers and executives is the amount of "territory" they control. The organization should want to encourage everyone to work toward the same goals, should it not? If, conversely, incentives are ineffective, if they are undeserved "perks," then they should be abolished for everyone. If incentives do not work, organizations are throwing away their money. If they do work, the organization should be consistent in its approach, determining what it wants to achieve and rewarding it powerfully.

Should the organization pay to get results? Incentive plans have been motivating senior managers in commercial industry for years. Why should the organization not fire up the middle managers too? The following proposal is open ended but varies with actual results. It pays only after 1 year of sustained and demonstrated savings. This plan is simple, fair, and proportional to the improvement in performance. The goal is to reward managers who cut costs and keep them down. Almost anyone can cut costs for a few weeks or even a few months, but permanent reductions are a different matter entirely. Sometimes this happens by accident—vacancies from maternity leave or illness, unexpected terminations, and the like. These are short term and quickly reverse. What the organization seeks is sustainable savings, a permanent change in the way managers conduct business. If they are capable of doing that, administration ought to send a reward their way to encourage them.

An incentive plan does not guarantee that all managers will earn a bonus. Administration should be delighted if everyone takes part, but there is no guarantee, or even expectation, that all managers would earn a reward. Over time, most managers might well find ways to become more efficient. All managers should be engaged to research, conceptualize, strategize, and implement. Having an incentive plan in place beforehand makes it more likely that managers will eagerly participate.

For the incentive calculation, department expenses would exclude any depreciation, interest, or bad debt charges from cost center reports, if they appear there at all. What remains is a good measure of what is under the department manager's direct control. Figure 5.2 is an example of what cost reduction with a program like this means to the organization. For simplicity, operating revenue is otherwise untouched so that the forecasted net operating margin can be calculated. The actual computation would apply to each department, using its own specific costs and units of service.

From the example in the Figure 5.2, compared with today, reducing "controllable" expenses by 6% would send $6.8 million more directly to the bottom line, lifting operating income to $9.3 million from the current $2.5 million and increasing operating

---

The *Triple Your Money Back* program: the manager's percentage salary bonus is triple that of the percentage cost reduction per unit achieved in his area year over year (excluding depreciation, interest, and bad debt expense, if any). The current year is the base year. A 6% decrease in department expenses per unit, for example, would earn the manager and eighteen percent bonus.

---

margins to 7.4% from 2.0%. If sustained for five years, such a margin would generate a 22% long-term incentive bonus for senior management as well so that everyone pulls together (7.4 − 2.0 × 4

= 21.6%). That is a great return on investment by anyone's yard-stick. Furthermore, suppose that volume and revenue growth were not constant as they are in the illustration. If revenue and volume were to grow over the year, and managers held the line on expenses, or even increased them slower than their volume growth, there would be an incentive bonus waiting for them. Organizations that have put together 5-year forecasts know the tremendous growth potential on the bottom line from restraining per-unit cost growth. In any event, the organization should approach this as a creative experiment in which it costs nothing to find the answer.

The value of using percentage reduction in expenses per unit as the performance measure is that it is immediately relevant to the department manager's area of influence. Year-over-year comparison means that purely temporary improvements are not rewarded, only those of a lasting or permanent nature. The incentive is proportional to both existing salaries and the value to the organization, producing twelve times as much as paid in incentives. If a department did not improve its operating position, the organization would pay nothing.

How to do the Calculations:

Controllable Expense: controllable expense per APD times adjusted patient days.

Controllable Expense per APD: today's controllable expense per APD less percentage decrease.

Cost of Bonus: percentage bonus multiplied by total manager salaries.

Net Value to Hospital: percentage reduction in controllable expense per APD, times three.

Return on Bonus: Net value to hospital divided by cost of bonus.

Dollars in Thousands (Except Where Noted)				
		Today	Hospital in 1 Year		
Expenses per Unit	Adjusted Patient Days (APD)	60,000	60,000	60,000	60,000
	Net Operating Revenue	125,000	125,000	125,000	125,000
	Interest, Depreciation, Bad Debt	10,000	10,000	10,000	10,000
	Controllable Expense*	112,500	108,000	105,750	103,500
	Net Operating Income	**2,500**	**7,000**	**9,250**	**11,500**
	Operating Margin	2.0%	5.6%	7.4%	9.2%
	Controllable Expense per APD (Whole $)	1,875	1,800	1,763	1,725
	Reduction in Expense per APD	0.0%	4.0%	6.0%	8.0%
Incentive Package	Total Manager Salaries	3,000	3,090	3,090	3,090
	Percentage Bonus	NA	12.0%	18.0%	24.0%
	Cost of Bonus	NA	371	556	742
	Net Value to Hospital	NA	4,500	6,750	9,000
	Return on Bonus	NA	12:1	12:1	12:1

* excluding interest, depreciation, bad debt

Figure 5.2. Cost reduction impact.

If a department did improve its performance, the organization would pay the bonus from a portion of the savings. Under an incentive plan like this, bonuses are more like a return on investment.

Of course, a health care organization could play with the "triple" formula. It might include an inflation allowance in the baseline cost for the current year, or use a different number for the multiplier. Whether it is made more or less generous, it should not be watered down to insignificance. When a department manager cuts $300,000 a year off his operating expenses, which is possible in a large, busy department, then the organization should give correspondingly big incentive bonuses. Instead of giving a gift coupon to the cafeteria, how about giving a car in the employee lot (donated from a local dealer)? Why not make a big splash and celebrate?

Are such savings achievable? No one can realistically know in advance. It is often surprising to find out how much discretion managers have. Today, they may devote considerable energy to increasing their labor pool, but with an incentive plan (and a push from productivity standards), they might direct their energy to eliminating valueless tasks, unnecessary reports, and other busy-work. For example, J. Philip Lathrop, in *Restructuring Health Care* (1994), estimated that about 50% of all labor organization-wide is devoted to clerical duties: 30% to scheduling, and 20% to scheduling transportation. Is there a better way?

There is a second benefit to the *Triple Your Money Back* plan. The inability of unsuccessful managers to earn large bonuses, when their colleagues are doing so, may lead them to voluntarily search for employment elsewhere, increasing the talent pool of the organization as a whole. In some other industries, the worst performing managers are continually rooted out. For the good of the organization, there must be some way to attract and retain talent while eliminating those who do not make the "cut." The advantage of this system is that it raises the competency of the whole organization without coercion, probation, and warnings. Under-performing managers would tend to weed *themselves* out.

The subject of incentives always raises issues of fairness: Some managers have more opportunity to reduce their costs than others do. Some managers grew their budgets every year while others held the line on their expenses, creating unequal savings opportunities. It follows that a few may be rewarded who perform well now but did not perform in the past. Why should those who took advantage in the past be rewarded for simply doing what others have always done? Why should those who have behaved responsibly in the past find their bonus opportunities reduced compared to their irresponsible peers?

These thoughts are all legitimate. All the same, the organization cannot be on a quest for social justice. It cannot right all of the wrongs of the past. So what if people earn different rewards? Results are what count. In business, as in life, no one has equal ability, and nothing is perfectly fair. The organization has to start somewhere, and it would be wrong to do nothing just to avoid uneven outcomes. The bigger outrage is that it is flagrantly unfair to burden many dedicated and capable people with having to subsidize the incompetent few. A balanced incentive plan can begin to right that problem.

The purpose of incentives is to stimulate exploration, discovery, and achievement. Does the organization want uninspired, underperforming managers to improve? Does it want to encourage outstanding performance from everyone, whatever their present circumstances? Anything else is a vote for mediocrity that will plague the organization for years. If an organization is only as good as the caliber of its people, then it ought to do something innovative, even courageous, to produce a company culture of star performers.

CONSEQUENCES

In the previous section, two incentive plans for rewarding superior performance were proposed that would help pull the organization higher. One plan was for executives, the other for department managers. Logically, if these plans have *any effect* on motivation and action, then the organization must benefit, for any organization is nothing more than the actions of all of its employees. If hurdles are removed, establishing the environment necessary for motivation to flourish, then that is exactly what the organization should witness. With the right organizational structure, some managers could achieve true superiority in their industry. Conversely, if administration merely expects managers to achieve standard, they will tend to stop at that point and progress no further. Many managers can do better than standard, and it only takes a few exceptional ones to lift the whole organization. With the help of incentives, the organization is poised to capitalize on great opportunities.

What then should happen when managers consistently and willfully miss their standard? Generally, organizations are somewhat reluctant to discipline poorly performing managers, particularly if there are lingering suspicions that budgets and standards are not realistic, little more than a dream. By exercising care when implementing the new productivity program, however, from analysis to negotiation to simplified monitoring, something very realistic and achievable can be produced. With such a solid foundation, there should be no reason to hesitate enforcing the program. The purpose of sanctions is to help motivate managers to meet established targets, while systematically weeding out poor performers if need be.

The problem has been twofold: no clear and explicit rules to hold managers accountable for meeting standards and, other than a general rule to observe the budget, no clear productivity policy spelling out who should be disciplined, what form it should take, and under what circumstances it should be administered. Although simple in essence—define minimum expectations and prescribe remedies—drafting the actual productivity policy presents a challenge. It has to be administered fairly, everyone must understand what is expected, and adequate resources must be made available to assist any faltering managers. It must be humane. The goal is not to fire managers, but help them perform to at least the minimum expectations of the organization.

Today, when managers do not obey their labor budgets, administration might raise a big fuss and hold special meetings. Analysts sum the negative variances and observe the results with alarm. The president might deliver a speech about the importance of adhering to budget targets. It might be perceived, as coined by Shakespeare, as full of sound and fury, signifying nothing. After all the bluster, the meetings, and other activities exhaust themselves, it almost always boils down to this: either there will be some sort of layoff or hiring freeze, or administration will wait a while longer and see if things start to look up. Many organizations have allowed themselves to be distracted and swayed by passing concerns.

- Budgets are often confusing and arbitrary, representing little more than an optimistic scenario fashioned after the first draft did not "pencil out."

- Goals can change from month to month, and pressing problems come and go.

- The *crisis du jour* consumes everyone's energy. Fires are doused, and stability returns (or the "crisis" is an over-reaction to a temporary anomaly and resolves by itself).

- Productivity control and monitoring is chaotic or ineffectual. Once the organization is forced to deal with escalating costs, it may over-react with freezes and layoffs, unwittingly planting the seeds for the next harvest of financial turmoil.

Nothing is more important to an organization's survival than control of its labor productivity. If the organization is prepared to reward superior performance, must it not also do something to discourage substandard management? As discussed in Chapter 3, the organization must establish the primacy of individual, not collective, responsibility. Collective responsibility is a meaningless term and unworkable in practice. The time has now come for the organization to define what poor management is and specify in writing what it is going to do about it. After all the work that has been accomplished, all the careful planning required to get to this stage, it must be made clear that meeting standard is not optional, and consistent failure to meet standard is grounds for dismissal. This will create the new culture of accountability.

This book developed a logical and fair set of principles for managers and executives. Now it is time to articulate the rules. First, a recap of the program to this point:

- Historical productivity for each department was analyzed in a consistent manner over several years. A target, or standard, was developed for each department. An analyst or consultant met with each of the department managers to discover if there was any reason why managers might not be able to meet their preliminary standard. When legitimate reasons were presented, such as an addition to department functions, the standard was altered to capture any adjustments.

- Departments could be either variable with workload volume or fixed, but not both. Managers chose which alternative best fit their operations.

- Department managers were granted unconditional hiring authority, including the right to determine skill mix in the interests of overall cost effectiveness (so long as they observed their cost per unit standard).

- The monitoring report format allowed quick and effective tracking of actual results against standard. The report mirrored the original productivity analysis; it made no "translations" from the analysis.

- The normal time reporting intervals were lengthened from the typical bi-weekly frequency to monthly and quarterly reporting in order to allow for temporary statistical fluctuations. This revealed true, underlying performance.

The organization cannot be constantly embroiled in basic productivity problems. There must be some firm bedrock principles to which it can safely anchor. It should not be deterred, retreating to familiar practices and procedures if it has some small difficulties in the first few months of the program. The old philosophies and policies yielded the old, unsatisfactory results.

The disposition against action until there is no other choice is all too common. Problems and opportunities are examined in excruciating detail, putting off a decision, and then everyone has to come to a consensus. Although this is sometimes a good thing—it avoids many mistakes—it also lets small problems escalate. The time to reach a consensus is before a crisis, not after. By deciding on a course of action in advance, the organization has the luxury of time, deliberation, thought, articulation, and communication on its side. By identifying the root causes of financial problems before they arise, it can act before there is a problem.

It is of the utmost importance for managers to perform their duties to the expectations of the organization. It is enough to set realistic standards and allow managers to achieve them. If they are not allowed to exercise personal responsibility for their actions and results, then administrators have to entertain any excuse, any rationale, as valid. The program outlined in this book removes most excuses as valid reasons for not meeting basic productivity standards, and allows for most contingencies. Aside from something truly out of managers' control, is there anything left? Even with a firm set of rules and principles that everyone agrees to observe, there still must be some discretion in the rulebook for rare, unforeseen events. The official productivity policy coming up leaves this final question to the discretion of executives. It is neither possible nor desirable to eliminate discretion. Instead, unlimited discretion can be reined in a bit, providing a proper place and time for its exercise.

Interestingly, a side effect of the incentive plan proposed earlier would also occur with the introduction of consequences: the changing culture may lead some managers to voluntarily search for employment somewhere else, a place where they do not stress accountability. When those who are willing to step up and be accountable replace managers who quit, it will have the effect of increasing the organization's talent pool.

How to Draft an Effective Productivity Policy

It is essential that an official policy be drafted and adopted so that the organization can be managed by principle, not by exception. With a written policy, it is much more likely that the executive team will follow through. Without it, everything will gradually become a matter of discretion for the testimonial committee once again, and the whole program will fall apart. The organization should not expend the effort and time it takes to develop, communicate, and implement standards if it is not absolutely committed to following through. This is not a good time for equivocation. Administration will have to muster the resolve to carry out the productivity program to its logical conclusion, and that is not easy. This means that managers who do not perform have to be removed. There is no way around that. The organization cannot tolerate poor management unless it is willing to risk the whole enterprise. Would it not be better to deal with any problems early when the price is reasonably low than wait until the cost is much higher?

Once the productivity policy is firmly entrenched, it will cease to become an issue. Once administration follows through the first time, the next time will not be for a long while; paradoxically, the existence of a productivity policy means that it seldom needs to be used. Just having it in place, ready when necessary, will be enough. Managers will respect the rules and the productivity policy will very seldom need to be followed to the end. It will simply become normal operating procedure.

Six Principles of an Effective Productivity Policy

The best policies are brief. These six principles can be used to draft a productivity policy that will keep the organization on track.

1. Who is responsible? Who has authority? Who monitors and reviews?

2. For what are they responsible? What happens if standards are not met?

3. When will performance be measured? What time period will be used?

4. Where will this take place?

5. How will performance be measured?

6. Why is the organization doing this? What is the purpose?

Here is one official policy that covers the above points:

Senior management has to make available adequate resources and expertise to assist managers to meet their responsibilities. Nevertheless, meeting productivity standards is properly the responsi-

Department managers are responsible for meeting their departmental productivity standards as established by the hospital. These standards are subject to change when circumstances warrant. Such standards consist of productive hours per unit of service and productive salaries per unit of service. In the case of "fixed" departments, those not on a variable workload measurement, such standards consist of total productive hours and total productive salaries. Consistent, long-term failure to meet these standards may be grounds for dismissal.

bility of each manager, who may employ such resources at his or her own discretion. Financial planning and performance are essential elements of management jobs.

Having decided what the organization wants to achieve and how it is going to accomplish that goal, the official policy can be simple and straightforward.

Establishing the Proper Limits

How much leeway should be given to managers to comply with standard? If a manager's performance were a bit worse than standard, would that be an infraction? The organization has to be reasonable about compliance, but at the same time, it cannot afford to be indulgent. If the labor budget for the organization is $100 million, for example, and it tolerates missing standards by 3%, then it exposes the organization to $3 million in cost overruns. That might be its entire annual net income! The organization has to decide this for itself, but a good guideline would be no more than 1%, which gives some measure of "forgiveness," yet does not expose the organization to undue financial risk. This means, in practice, that the standard is an upper limit—a ceiling, not a floor. There is a little room for measurement variability, but not much.

The next thing to decide is how to apply the tolerance limit. Remember that there are two main performance standards, hours per unit and cost per unit. Should the organization apply the 1% tolerance, as suggested previously, to both hours and cost per unit? Some might say that cost is more important and hours are secondary. Although that has a large measure of truth, over time a department could run into a problem when employees come and go at different wage rates. Although that might be normal and explainable, it would become difficult to account for—except in terms of the number of hours worked. On the other hand, if the focus is exclusively on hours worked, then the unintended consequence of encouraging unwanted skill mix inflation is real. In practice, it is best to interpret one statistic by reference to the other. Therefore, it seems best to monitor both hours and dollars, and apply the same rules to each. Exceptions can always be made later if the opportunity arises. After all, if a department submits a plan to increase its number of hours, yet reduce total cost, then that should certainly be evaluated as a reasonable request, perhaps altering the standards to account for the new arrangement.

Keep It Public

In the interest of keeping productivity a hot topic, it is a good idea to have a monthly meeting of all department managers and executives to review the latest monthly, quarterly, and year-to-date productivity results. The idea is to keep everyone informed of the dollar impact each department is having on the organization, whether positive or negative. No manager wants to see his department's poor performance on display, but everyone wants to see his department's strong performance on display. The names of the departments can be hidden, but that is not recommended. There is nothing wrong with a little peer pressure to keep managers and executives motivated. If everyone is supposed to be in this together, then everyone has a need to know, and nothing should be hidden.

In addition to the monthly productivity review, senior management should monitor compliance to productivity standards in a quarterly review through a productivity committee it creates. Instead of taking testimony, its functions are financial oversight, procedure revisions, and enforcing compliance to written policy (refer back to the section titled Don't Take Testimony, and Rules for Changing Standards in Chapter 3).

Productivity Committee Procedure

Variable departments measure performance to standard against the monthly cost center reports, under the "Better/Worse than Standard" column (see the section titled Format of the Productivity Report in Chapter 4). The standard and total budget is the same for fixed departments. If a manager's performance against *either* the hours or salary standard were unfavorable by more than 1% for the last quarter, a written explanation and correction plan would be submitted to the vice president. If performance against *both* hours and salary standard were unfavorable by more than 1% for the last quarter, vice presidents would discuss their correction plans with the productivity committee and the affected manager. The committee would follow up to ensure compliance by the end of the next quarter.

The vice president's role is to develop action plans, monitor progress, and counsel managers on performance improvement. If performance lagged behind standard in one quarter, managers would be required to make it up in the following quarter, so that their two-quarter performance is within 1% of standard. That gives managers a half-year to get things on track.

Parting Company

In this scenario, the productivity committee followed the procedure fairly, and the department's performance did not improve after two quarters. What would happen then?

In the absence of extenuating circumstances, if department performance had not materially improved after two quarterly reviews by the Productivity Committee, it would be time to prepare for the manager's departure. The committee would present the following options if there were no extenuating circumstances prohibiting a manager from making the necessary changes, or if the committee decided that performance would be unlikely to improve given time. If a manager cannot, or will not, improve his or her department's performance to standard there can be no other option but termination. Administrators would have no choice but to prevent costly problems from escalating and make room for someone else to try managing the department. If not, it would leave the door open to a breakdown and layoffs down the road. Better to lose a few managers than many more employees. Staff should not be penalized for poor management when the situation is preventable. Termination can take three forms:

1. *Voluntary resignation with 90 days paid severance:* Ninety days of pay is generous, and helps to soften the blow. The goal is not to punish the manager, but to move him or her out so that someone else can move in. A voluntary resignation also preserves the manager's career options.

2. *Ninety-day probationary period in which to meet productivity standards, with forfeiture of ninety days' severance pay:* If the manager is successful at meeting standard, then probation would be terminated and everything resumes as normal. If the manager is not successful, involuntary or voluntary termination ensues, with only the normal amount of severance pay per existing organization policy.

3. *Transfer to a new position within the organization:* It is entirely possible that the manager is extremely capable, just not in the present position. If there is a vacant position suitable for his or her talents, he or she should be given every encouragement to stay and take on a different position.

The organization must take great pains that these options are arranged in secret so that no one is publicly humiliated. No one on either side of the table wants to go through this process. It is painful and disruptive; nevertheless, the organization must exercise its responsibilities. The intent is not to make an example of anyone, only to fix the situation. People will realize soon enough what is happening. Administration should ensure that these proceedings are conducted with dignity and compassion.

In all probability, only a small minority of managers would get to this stage. Which of the three options is most attractive? That depends on whether the manager wishes to continue at the organization. The important thing is to look out for the good of the organization. Certainly, administration should be willing to accommodate individuals, but not to the extent of sacrificing the organization's finances. Certain responsibilities come with the job, they are not new, and they may not be ignored. Virtually every management job description says something about financial responsibility and supporting the organization's financial goals. What is new is that the organization is insisting that these responsibilities be made real.

SUMMARY

Chapter 2 proposed a logical and clear analytical approach that gave a convincing and rational set of practical recommendations that could be implemented immediately. Chapter 3 turned to implementation. The case was made that the usual approval process is dysfunctional and counter-productive; that the signatures, signoffs, and other procedures designed to encourage thrift actually increase labor costs throughout the organization. To fix this problem, department managers must have autonomy, provided they are held to a firm standard, thereby allowing control of the outcome, not the process. Defining exactly what the organization wants to achieve in advance, then delegating and authorizing those responsible for its attainment, allows the productivity initiative to succeed.

The organization must address the rationale for asking people to change. What reason is there to improve? The motivational theme that may well be most effective would explain the purpose of profit in a meaningful way that relates to people, their motivations, their passions, and their purpose. All who contribute to the welfare of the organization and its mission, and those who benefit from it, should find the experience enriching.

Without the effect of incentives to motivate people to exceed expectations or of consequences for not delivering, implementation will fall well short of the potential within reach. It does no good to lay down the rules and not follow through on them. It is critical that the health care organization establishes a long-term maintenance program to prevent sliding back to the same place it was before. Although labor standards define the *minimum* performance an organization will accept, an effective incentive plan motivates managers to *exceed* their targets.

A common objection to incentive plans is that managers will be rewarded for cutting service and quality to save money. Although overblown, it does raise a valid concern. If the organization needs to overcome an unfounded fear that incentive plans would cause harm, a link should be made between cost and quality, so that one is not obtained at the expense of the other. The ultimate goal of the organization is turning out the best medical outcomes at the lowest cost. If quality can be defined and measured for every department, it will be known if managers have achieved their quality goals.

The organization ought to structure management jobs to reward the successful as it disciplines the marginal performers. Having no incentives or consequences unintentionally punishes the successful and ambitious, and rewards those who shun initiative. An intelligent system of incentives and consequences has three components: variable management compensation with large upside potential, recognition and reward for outstanding performance, and departure of the incompetent.

An official written productivity policy removes most discretion, arbitrariness, and politics from decision making, substituting principle, rule, and procedure in their stead. The six principles of an effective policy answer the questions who, what, when, where, how, and why. Paradoxically, the existence of an official, plainly written productivity policy means that it seldom needs to be followed to the end. Just having it in place, ready when necessary, will be enough.

THE POLITICS
OF PRODUCTIVITY

Decision-making at health care organizations tends to be rather deliberate. Practice and custom often require that a near consensus be reached among various parties, some with competing agendas. An important force with which to be reckoned, the medical staff does not even work for the organization. On the other hand, consensus means that once a decision is reached to improve productivity, people will most likely support it to the best of their abilities.

At the outset the chance of encountering opposition to productivity improvement is likely to be high in some quarters. From past experience, people can feel threatened and uneasy. Then again, it is not a foregone conclusion that disagreement will be overwhelming. The best approach is to come equipped with a thoughtful response for all parties so that cooperation can be obtained.

Voluntary cooperation is based on the principle of exchange—one gives something of greater value to the recipient than oneself and receives something of greater value to oneself than to the recipient.

"EVEN IF YOU'RE ON THE RIGHT TRACK, YOU'LL GET RUN OVER IF YOU JUST SIT THERE."
—WILL ROGERS

Cooperation offers something to each of the participants. Neutralizing the politics of productivity involves understanding the organization's constituencies and taking up their concerns by offering them something they value in exchange for their willing participation.

MEDICAL STAFF

Unless doctors have some equity in the organization, the reality is that they have no direct financial interest in improving productivity. In fact, they quite literally have no interest in supply utilization, clinical benchmarking, or any other project motivated solely by finances, a reality that has frustrated many organizations as they seek to improve their cost structures.

Administration realizes that medical staff drives cost, but doctors cannot be controlled, at least not in the same manner as employees. Is the nature of the relationship between doctor and organization a bad thing? If the organization cannot compel, then it must rely on collaboration. This is probably a good thing. What do doctors want from their organizations? The list usually reads something like this:

- *Exceptional clinical service and support:* Doctors take direct care of their patients, but they need the support of highly skilled and dedicated clinical staff. They do not appreciate obstacles to patient care, and they are ready to take their business elsewhere if there is a more convenient, effective alternative. They use the organization as a kind of workshop, where the best tools and materials are expected to be at their disposal. The organization tends to think of patients as "theirs," but patients really "belong" to the doctors. The doctors are the organization's primary customers, and they can (and should) be demanding.

- *Seamless coordination of services:* The organization may move patients from department to department for cost reasons, as, for example, moving patients from the lab to radiology or from one ward to another. Everyone accepts some level of scheduling and transportation, but this is for the convenience and cost of the organization, not the patient or doctor. Doctors want the various services for their patients delivered at the right time, every time.

- *Easy patient access into, and out of, the hospital:* Scheduling and then admitting a patient is not always an easy process. Arranging for on-time discharge is also challenging. Hospitals have been getting better in recent years as they become more responsive to customer demands and cost pressures. Still, the easier the process becomes, the better it is for the doctor.

- *Highly responsive, customer-focused administrators:* Doctors rightly consider themselves the organization's customer. Whether they ask for convenient block scheduling times or to perform cutting-edge procedures, they expect administration to be highly responsive to their needs.

- *A bare minimum of bureaucracy:* Doctors do not like to hassle with multiple layers of management, to attend meetings with no clear purpose, or to experience undue delays any more than anyone else. They want to take care of each patient in the most efficient manner and move on to the next patient.

- *First-rate technology:* Advances in medical technology allow doctors to get more accuracy and speed than ever before. Equipment advances improve medical outcomes. Doctors expect the organization to keep up with technology.

These goals are also found to some extent in every organization's mission statement, an expression of its core values. Attaining these objectives, however, requires money. If the organization is going broke, improving clinical quality and purchasing advanced medical technology is virtually impossible. Doctors know this perfectly well; they are in business and they understand the importance of profit. Therefore, the organization should offer a trade: if physicians help lower costs, the organization helps fund the physicians' goals. One way that physicians can help lower costs is by participating in productivity improvement initiatives or simply by not opposing them. Doctors will not offer opposition if they believe that the organization must reduce its labor costs and that the program the organization is advancing offers the best way to do it. If these are mutual objectives, both parties can prosper by working toward the same ends.

Beyond that, the medical staff's chief desire is likely to be that cost reduction not hurt quality or service. The organization shares this desire as well. The productivity program in this book is laid out in such a way that quality need not be affected, as the case studies in the appendix make clear (also see the section titled Quality Standards in Chapter 5). Service enhancements that departments have made can be preserved while still improving overall organization productivity. This was the purpose of meeting with department managers individually, as outlined in Chapter 2.

Some medical directors may want to work together with their department managers as the organization unveils its productivity improvement program. After all, requirements concerning productivity and budgeting are in the standard medical director job description. If medical directors are not so inclined, the organization and its managers should to take it upon themselves to keep the medical staff informed of progress.

LABOR UNIONS

What do labor unions want for their members? If the organization understands these desires, it will be in a better position to offer something in return for the unions' cooperation.

- *Job security:* Unions act to preserve jobs for their members. In some industries, they have even been able to preserve jobs that are obsolete or of marginal value. Nevertheless, if employers have to cut labor costs to survive, the best that unions can do is delay the inevitable.

- *Higher wages:* Unions are monopoly labor collectives; and work to ensure higher wages for their members than would probably be earned in a comparable non-union shop.

- *Good working conditions:* Employees want managers to respect their opinions, to let them have a say about any decisions that affect them, and help them work in a friendly atmosphere where they can make a positive contribution.

These things are desired by all employees, unionized or not. The satisfaction of these demands improves job satisfaction, builds morale, creates excellent service, and brings down turnover and absenteeism. In turn, these lead to lower training and recruitment costs, reduced worker's compensation claims, and less overtime and registry—the costs of low job satisfaction. These outcomes are extremely desirable to the organization.

Once again, the organization can propose a trade to secure the unions' cooperation (or at least their forbearance): if the union will help raise productivity, greater job security for everyone will result. Except in an unforeseen fiscal emergency, there will be virtually no cause for layoffs, since the organization will have achieved better productivity. Perhaps there will be more available for wage increases or at least the ability to meet market rate (meeting the market is also important to reduce the costs listed previously). Administration can explain its sincere desire to work with its unions, shunning layoffs for a smoother transition—one without strikes or headlines. In this regard, administration would like the same outcomes as the union.

Understanding what unions want for their members allows the organization to offer something of value to the unions in return for their support.

EXECUTIVES

Strangely enough, one of the most significant challenges to this program is the obstacle that executives may present. The difficulty arises as the consequence of moving authority from the executives to their department managers (see the section titled The New Deal in Chapter 3). While this places responsibility at the proper operating level for results, it also means that executives give up some control as their managers assume more autonomy.

Executives may be uncomfortable delegating their authority in this important area. Promoted based on their extensive experience and good judgment, executives may very well want to keep their power intact. In principle, they may agree that authority should be pushed down the ladder. They may agree that managers should take more responsibility for the operations of their departments. In practice, however, they may not be ready to give up control. People accustomed to exercising authority may not readily abandon it.

At Centennial Hospital, Shirley, a relatively new senior vice president, voiced strong opposition to the productivity plan. She said, "In my professional opinion, this program will not work. Managers will not be able to handle it. They won't be that responsible and they can't be trusted with more authority." Such a sentiment highlights the political issues of dealing with control and authority moving around the organization in ways that not everyone may welcome. Obviously, such opposition in high quarters cannot stand and have the program move forward. It had to be addressed quickly, and after much spirited debate among the executive team, the President stepped in and made the final call to move ahead, saying "Productivity is the number one priority this year. We must do this."

This vignette underscores the vital importance of leadership. A successful long-term implementation must address these issues in the following ways.

1. Executives should be encouraged to shift their focus and apply their experience to strategic planning, not the micro-management of department operations.

2. Executives' workload will lighten as they delegate responsibility to their managers. That should be an attractive prospect for those who complain about their long working hours.

3. Executives need to recognize their vital oversight role in the new scheme: ensuring results in accord with the organization's productivity policy (see Chapter 5). Managers will need their support, especially through the early period of implementation.

The president or CEO must demonstrate commitment to the new system, providing leadership through the critical early months of implementation and beyond. Total commitment to the new system is so crucial that it can hardly be overstated.

DEPARTMENT MANAGERS

Just as some executives may resist granting more autonomy to managers, some managers may not be eager to secure more independence for themselves. Autonomy comes at a price: with new authority come new obligations. To managers unaccustomed to such focused accountability, it may seem a bit daunting. The complexity of the budgeting and productivity system may have confounded efforts to increase accountability, or the approval process may have shifted the weight of responsibility to others, but all that is no more.

The trade offered to managers is clear: managers take responsibility for meeting standard, and the organization removes all obstacles to doing so. In other words, it grants the authority to act. Gone are the hassles of convincing others of one's case, the demeaning testimonials, approvals, and countersignatures. Gone is the needless convolution and incomprehensibility of productivity management. Even the budgeting process can be made remarkably easier and quicker by budgeting from standard, not the last 6–12 months of actual labor. Because most of the organization's expenses are labor costs, cleaning up this area makes the whole budget easier, quicker, and more accurate. For managers used to the hassle of formulating and negotiating budgets, the prospect of a budget process that is fair, quick, and easy should be very welcome.

All that said, significant resistance by department managers is unlikely. They are used to managing their labor resources, and the program in this book simply replaces the current regime. What this program offers is freedom with limits, and the advantages should be promoted to managers until they get used to the idea.

THE BOARD

Serving on the board are the "insiders" (members of senior management) and the "outsiders" (business people, community leaders, and perhaps a few health care professionals). Although the outsiders provide a valuable point of view, they generally know relatively little about health care provider management. They determine the financial goals and strategic direction of the organization, leaving the specific techniques to be employed as the prerogative of senior management.

Regarding productivity, the outsiders on the board will be concerned about three things, that: 1) the plan is logical and sound, 2) it has a reasonable chance of success, and 3) the plan is fair. The program meets all these criteria, but it has to be properly explained to the board. When management promotes a coherent productivity plan, the board will likely welcome it as an indispensable tactic to control costs. It is up to management to make the case that labor costs must be trimmed down, and that this is the best way to do it.

PRODUCTIVITY FOR THE LONG TERM

A truly successful productivity improvement program in the long term is one that seeks to raise the general level of commitment and motivation toward organizational goals. Chapter 5 advances the position that action directed toward the achievement of goals is mostly a matter of incentives and disincentives, and that the great problem at many organizations is the absence of explicit rewards for achievement as well as consequences for poor performance. Administration would do well to go a little further by setting a superior motivational tone throughout the organization to energize long-term productivity management. Ideally, explicit incentives and disincentives would be supplemented with a coordinated campaign to raise the general level of motivation in all employees to very high levels. Clearly, this would be a most important job for the executive team. Motivation depends on the individual and his or her circumstances. Figure 6.1 summarizes the list of motivators and de-motivators from the most popular motivational theories.

How might the organization increase motivation? As with most things in business, it all comes from the top. The character of an organization is a reflection of the characters of its executives. A senior administration modeling trust and respect; recognizing achievement; being open, available, and brutally honest; and showing genuine concern for the welfare of employees would natu-

Top Workplace Motivators	Top Workplace De-motivators
• Recognition	• Low wages
• Meaningful responsibilities	• Job insecurity
• Stimulating and challenging work	• Low influence and status
• Freedom to be creative	• Little recognition
• Achievement	• Little challenge
• Influence and status	• Little freedom to be creative
• Learning and career developments	• Inferior working conditions
• Exceptional working relationships	• Poor working relationships

Figure 6.1. The top motivators and de-motivators from the most popular motivational theories.

rally engender superb motivation and commitment throughout the organization. Having good intentions and feelings is not enough—these qualities must be made readily visible to all. Setting clear expectations for performance matched with appropriate incentives and consequences, removing unnecessary obstacles, and creating accountability up and down the line are giant leaps in the right direction.

What is the payoff? Aside from a great work environment that benefits both employees and patients in numerous ways, the list includes improved job satisfaction and customer service, lower turnover and absenteeism, followed by lower training and recruitment costs, and less overtime and registry.

SUMMARY

The chance of encountering opposition to productivity improvement is likely to be high in some quarters. The best approach is to come equipped with a thoughtful response for all parties so that cooperation can be obtained. Cooperation is based on the principle of exchange, giving and taking in equal measure. The major players in the organization are the doctors, labor unions, executives, managers, and the board. Neutralizing the politics of productivity involves understanding the organization's constituencies and taking up their concerns by offering them something of value in exchange for their cooperation.

Doctors want exceptional clinical service and support; seamless coordination of organization services; easy patient access into, and out of, the hospital or clinic; responsive, customer-focused administrators; a minimum of bureaucracy; and first-rate technology. The organization wants these things too. If physicians help lower costs by supporting improved productivity, the organization helps fund the physicians' goals.

Labor unions want job security, higher wages, and good working conditions. These things ought to improve job satisfaction, customer service, turnover, and absenteeism, followed by lower training and recruitment costs, and less overtime and registry. These outcomes are extremely desirable to the organization. If the union will help raise productivity, greater job security for everyone will result, without layoffs.

As executives give up some control to their managers, problems may surface. Executives may be uncomfortable delegating their authority. A successful long-term implementation addresses this problem by encouraging executives to shift their focus from micro-management to strategic planning, oversight, and guidance. They will benefit from seeing long hours become shorter. On the other side of the coin, some managers may not be eager to secure more independence; autonomy comes at a price, but it has its advantages too. The arrangement: managers take responsibility for meeting standard, and the organization removes all obstacles to doing so.

The board is mainly concerned with strategy, leaving the specific plans to be employed as senior management's prerogative. The board will only need to be satisfied that the productivity plan is logical and sound, that it will succeed, and that it is fair. It is up to management to make the case that labor costs must be cut, and that this is the best way to do it.

A truly successful productivity improvement program in the long term is one that seeks to raise the general level of commitment and motivation toward organizational goals. Ideally, explicit incentives and disincentives would be supplemented with a coordinated campaign to raise the general level of motivation. A senior administration modeling trust and respect, recognizing achievement, and showing concern for employee welfare would naturally engender superb motivation and commitment. This would make for a great work environment that benefits both employees and patients in numerous ways—including superior productivity.

CASE STUDIES

Real case studies represent a variety of different departments. Actual examples of situations and solutions help illustrate how to put concepts into practice. Discovering the root of the problem will usually dictate a logical course of action, and, in many cases, the required adjustments are relatively uncomplicated. The departments represented touch upon the main areas of the organization, including ancillary patient care, support services, and nursing. To protect confidentiality, some of the details have been disguised in the following three illustrations.

EMERGENCY ROOM

Small improvements in large departments offer more savings than large improvements in small departments. This ER showed 2 years of successive productivity losses totaling more than 36,000 hours and $815,000 (see Figure A1). Although the department had grown

			Total Labor		Per Unit		Productivity Change	
	Unit of Service	Volume	Hours	Wages	Hours	Wages	Hours	Wages
2000	ER Visit	36,667	75,596	1,883,879	2.06	51.38	NA	NA
2001	ER Visit	43,656	112,905	2,471,231	2.59	56.61	(22,900)	(501,225)
2002	ER Visit	47,853	137,618	3,119,417	2.88	65.19	(13,859)	(314,135)
Three Year Performance		128,176	326,119	7,474,527	2.54	58.31	(36,758)	(815,360)

Figure A1. Performance of the emergency room.

over the years, its labor use had grown even faster, reaching 2.88 hours per visit. With *more volume,* this ER was getting *less efficient,* compounding the total losses.

A series of visits with the department manager ensued. The interviews revealed that the budget had grown because it was calculated from the last 6 months of actual staffing. Owing to confusion about the precise meaning of productivity, staffing control at the department level was lax, and effective executive oversight had gone astray. As the department kept staffing up, the budget "grandfathered" the increase and made it the new base for the coming year. This meant that productivity losses were made part of the next year's budget. In addition, whenever volume rose for any length of time, the manager had made regular, successful appeals to the Operations Committee for more fixed and variable staff. Adding fixed staff severed the connection to volume, making it easier to get committee approval. The variable staff requisitions were in excess of actual volume increases.

The rather large loss in hourly productivity multiplied by the sheer size of the department represented a huge savings potential, positioning the ER department at the very top of the savings opportunities list. Not surprisingly, the manager put up some resistance, explaining changes to department operations over the past 3 years that in her opinion invalidated the productivity analysis. Some of these changes were indeed material, while others were simply volume-related, for which the department would receive full credit. Recapturing the performance in 2000 would pose an analytical

problem, for there were a few changes in the department's responsibilities and functions that occurred mid-year that would complicate
the analysis. The major change taking place was the assumption of
housekeeping duties within the department. The addition of housekeeping staff actually was responsible for only a minor amount of
the change in productivity year over year.

Nevertheless, in the face of manager resistance in so large a department, a judgment call had to be made. Would it be better to go
through a detailed analysis and attempt to capture 100% of the opportunity, further deepening resistance, or compromise for the sake
of getting what would still represent large savings quickly? Another
important consideration: This manager was clearly an opinion
leader among her peers at the organization, and her department's
position at the head of the savings list is part of what made success
here crucial. Although the other managers at this organization
found the advantages of the productivity program attractive, this
manager was the sole opponent. If she could make it, resistance elsewhere would be much reduced (this proved the case). The path of
least resistance dictated that it would be better to give a little to get
a lot. Further productivity improvement could always be taken up
later.

In this case, the consultant-organization analyst team was well
aware that the average industry benchmark for ERs of this type was
2.1 hours per visit, further corroborating the analysis. The analyst
or consultant who conducts these productivity meetings must be
sure of these facts. Thus, despite resistance from the manager, there
was no principled reason not to establish the department's standard
at the 2001 level of 2.59 hours per visit. With their knowledge, a
reasonable compromise was reached that minimized the manager's
resistance: The standard was set at the 2001 level of 2.59 hours per
visit, for a calculated savings of more $300,000 annually.

The standard now set, the manager swiftly cooperated and
looked at staffing patterns in the department. She discovered that
staffing was highest on weekday afternoons, even though volume

subsided during that time. Overlapping shifts and prescheduled overtime contributed to the problem. After consulting her staff over the next 3 months, the manager virtually eliminated scheduled overtime and reduced overlapping shifts to a minimum. In 4 months, these changes drove the department's performance to a level much better than standard, saving $500,000 per year. Although hours were reduced for some workers, not a single layoff occurred.

The organization helped the effort by holding monthly presentations on the state of productivity. Every department's results were displayed for all to see. The same public forum was used to celebrate the success of the ER and the manager's capable leadership. Peer role models are critical to the effort.

DIETARY

Dietary is another large and visible function. In this case study, consulting dietitians and nutritionists were excluded from the analysis to make better comparisons, leaving only the kitchen. This analysis showed erratic staffing patterns. The department improved its productivity in 2001 and then took a step backward in 2002, costing the organization $124,000 in lost productivity (see Figure A2). The goal was to reverse this loss.

Several meetings with the manager revealed the issue. The department had lost several good employees, including a shift supervisor, and sought to hire replacements. The organization's hiring committee had deferred the request, leaving the manager to resort to temporary staffing and overtime to fill the gap. The former shift supervisor's role, which had not been delegated to someone else, was critical in monitoring staffing levels. Lax oversight and training problems showed up in productivity losses. The manager arranged

	Unit of Service	Volume	Total Labor		Per Unit		Productivity Change	
			Hours	Wages	Hours	Wages	Hours	Wages
2000	100 Meals Served	5,182	97,681	1,151,026	18.85	222.12	NA	NA
2001	100 Meals Served	6,670	97,515	1,173,470	14.62	175.93	28,215	339,531
2002	100 Meals Served	6,575	107,173	1,198,372	16.30	182.26	(11,047)	(123,523)
	Three Year Performance	18,427	302,369	3,522,868	16.41	191.18	17,168	216,008

Figure A2. Performance of the Dietary department.

to reduce excess staffing in exchange for permission to hire a few highly qualified replacements for the temporary workers and overtime. As this fit well within the proposed standard of 14.62 hours per 100 meals served, the manager would be free to make the change in order to return to the productivity performance of 2001. It was explained to the manager that he would not need permission to hire, so long as he observed the productivity standard established in 2001. This freedom to make the necessary changes proved most advantageous to secure the manager's cooperation. Once the productivity program was officially enacted, the manager hired a shift supervisor, and together they regained control of staffing, pushing the use of temporary and overtime staff down to reasonable levels. Productivity gradually improved to better than standard. Three months later, the manager's success was celebrated in the monthly manager's meeting.

Many managers will verify that registry and overtime workers are not as effective or productive as regular workers are. Pressed to produce savings, budget committees may unwittingly discourage the replacement of premium-time with straight-time workers. Paper savings are created when registry is categorized not as labor expense, but as a purchased service. If so, registry will not even appear in the organization's headcount statistics. It is vital that health care organizations aggregate all labor, of whatever type, into labor statistics for analysis and monitoring (emphasized in Chapter 2).

MOTHER/BABY UNIT

The goal for this unit was recapturing productivity of 7.68 hours per patient day in 2000 (see Figure A3). Reaching this goal would save $338,000 a year. The manager revealed that the organization had granted two clerical positions to cope with the paperwork and effect better discharge planning. The people had been hired, and the manager thought they were working very well. Such positions represent a definable service level improvement that the organization made a deliberate decision to achieve. Therefore, it was agreed that the department should operate at 7.68 hours per patient day and add to that the new positions added in 2001. This brought the standard to 8.01 hours per patient day, which still meant $238,000 in annual savings to the organization.

The manager wanted to check her department's staffing grid, which compares staffing levels in relation to patient census (see Figure A4). While the department's staffing grid produced hours per patient day that agreed with the proposed standard, investigation showed that evening and night shift supervisors regularly overrode the staffing grid, causing the department to perform less efficiently than in the past. Training on the proper use of the staffing grid and the importance of meeting standard solved the staffing issue.

Nursing units' staffing grids can serve as a convenient and useful adjunct to the productivity analysis. Occasionally, nursing units will deviate from their staffing grids with good cause. When this oc-

	Unit of Service	Volume	Total Labor Hours	Total Labor Wages	Per Unit Hours	Per Unit Wages	Productivity Change Hours	Productivity Change Wages
2000	Patient Days	11,343	87,081	2,179,585	7.68	192.15	NA	NA
2001	Patient Days	12,332	98,268	2,385,022	7.97	193.40	(3,594)	(87,230)
2002	Patient Days	12,168	107,004	2,668,329	8.79	219.29	(10,043)	(250,436)
Three Year Performance		35,843	292,353	7,232,936	8.16	201.79	(13,637)	(337,666)

Figure A3. Performance of the Mother/Baby Unit.

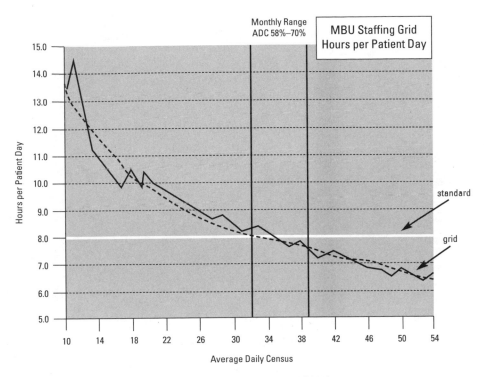

Figure A4.   Staffing grid for hours spent per patient in the Mother/Baby Unit (MBU).

curs too frequently, however, productivity suffers. Resetting the staffing grid, or observing the one already in place, is an important step to introduce staffing consistency for performance to standard over the long run.

GLOSSARY
OF TERMS

Accountability   Responsibility to someone for some activity; officially held to account for performance

Acuity   Generally refers to the severity of a patient's medical condition; also the amount or level of care needed by a patient corresponding to his or her medical condition

Administrative costs   Costs not directly related to, or in direct support of, the care of patients; a subset of *Overhead*

Agency worker   A temporary worker hired through an agency; synonymous with *Registry worker*

Authority   The ability and official authorization to implement appropriate actions as needed

Benchmarking   A systematic process for evaluating, comparing, and adopting industry practices recognized as best in class in order to reduce cost or enhance quality

Budget   An itemized summary of estimated or intended expenditures and revenues for a given period along with proposals for financing

Company culture   The predominating attitudes and behavior that characterize the functioning of an organization

Consequence   A remedy that logically or naturally follows from an unfavorable action or undesirable condition; something that prevents or discourages action, a deterrent

Controllable expenses   Total department expenses excluding depreciation, interest, or bad debt charges; a useful measure of what is under a department manager's direct control

Core-staffing schedule   Refers to the base level of staffing required on a unit by shift, also known as core coverage

Department manager   The person who controls department resources and expenditures and directs all administrative functions of a department

Discharge   An inpatient released from the hospital to his home or to another facility

Downsizing   See *Layoff*

Executive   Person or group having senior administrative or managerial authority in an organization, usually vice president or higher rank

Fixed costs   Costs that must be paid regardless of patient volume or revenues, including interest expense, rent, utilities, certain administrative costs, depreciation, and so forth; a part of *Overhead*

Fixed labor   Labor costs and hours that must be paid regardless of patient volume or revenues, at least in the short term (e.g., certain administrative costs)

Flexible budget   A recalculated budget that takes into account actual workload volumes, not budgeted volumes (i.e., flexible with actual volumes)

Float pool   An in-house group of employees who are directed to the particular departments in which they are needed (i.e., they "float" to those departments)

FTE   Full-time equivalent, equal to 2,080 hours per year, including vacation time, sick time, and holidays

Incentive   A positive motivational influence that induces action or motivates effort; an additional payment to managers as a means of increasing productivity

Industrial engineering   The application of scientific and mathematical principles to practical ends, such as the design, manufacture, and operation of efficient processes and systems

Labor expense   The sum of salaries, wages, temporary workers, registry workers, and overtime; may also include related employee benefits

Layoff   A mass termination of employees

Management engineering   The application of scientific and mathematical principles to productivity management

Master schedule   Prescribes the level of staffing for various patient volumes by shift

Nonproductive hours and costs   Hours and costs paid for vacation time, sick time, and holidays and sometimes training

On-call   A designation for a class of employees available to work as needed, often at odd hours, with minimum advance notice

Over-engineering   The engineering of a product, process, or system beyond the point of further utility or benefit

Overhead   Operating expenses excluding direct patient care and related support, such as billing costs, housekeeping, interest expense, depreciation, and administrative costs

Overtime   Working hours and wages in addition to those of a regular schedule, paid at premium wage rates

Paid hours   The sum of productive and nonproductive hours

Paid wages   The sum of productive and nonproductive wages

Patient day   The daily count of inpatients usually done at a set time (midnight) throughout the hospital

Power   The ability or official capacity to exercise control, authority

Productive hours and wages   Hours and wages spent working, excluding vacation time, sick time, and holidays and sometimes preservice or in-service training

Productivity   The amount of output per unit of labor input, expressed as hours or cost per unit of service

Productivity standard   A productivity measure or statistic that relates workload to staffing, expressed as hours or cost per unit of service; also called *Labor standard*

Reengineering   The examination and modification of a process to reconstitute it in a new form and the subsequent implementation of the new form

Registry worker   Worker (usually a nurse) hired through an outside agency

Responsibility   An obligation or duty that an individual assumes or takes upon him- or herself; the quality of being responsible

Rules   A prescribed direction for conduct; governing procedures

Skill mix   The average level of training, certification, and experience; the job classes or occupations of individuals in a department

Span of control   The number of employees (usually expressed as FTE) per manager

Step-variable   The term applied to the tendency for fixed staff to increase in irregular spurts or steps, not smoothly with increases in patient volume

Straight time   Regularly scheduled employee hours or wages excluding overtime, premium holiday pay, and so forth

Temporary worker   A worker hired from an outside agency whose duration is intended to be temporary, usually to fill in for employee absences and vacations or to work temporary jobs

Unit of service   A workload measure that describes a department's mission, its purpose, or its patients (e.g., patient days, visits, procedures, treatments, cases)

Variable costs   Costs that vary in direct proportion with workload volume

Variable labor   Labor hours and costs that vary in direct proportion with workload volume

Worked hours and wages   See *Productive hours and wages*

Workload volume or statistic   See *Unit of service*

INDEX

Page numbers followed by *f* indicate figures.

Absences, as indicator, 18
Accountability, 3, 78–84, 181
  and authority, 81–82
  budgetary, 83–84
  executive, 81–84
  individual, 78–81, 145
  and micromanagement, 107
  and responsibility, 78
  versus the Law of Unintended Consequences, 108–109
Acuity, 181
Adjustment factors, 32
Administrative costs, *see* Fixed/variable costs
Agency, *see* Registry
Analysis, 34–50
  categorizing, 35–43
  expectations, 45–46
  length of, 45, 58, 91–92, 97
  and transition to productivity program, 92–93
Authority, 181
  and accountability, 3, 81–82
  lack of, 3
  and responsibility, 78, 176–177

Benchmarking, 12f,, 181
  internal, 61–62,
  and labor standards, 10, 30–32
  and productivity programs, 11
"Best performers," *see* Benchmarking
Budgets, 182
  flexible, 2–3
  overreliance on, 2–3

Collaboration, and politics, 161–162, 169–171
  in the board of directors, 168
  in department managers, 165
  and executive leadership, 163, 168–169
  in labor unions, 164–165
  in medical staff, 162–164
Company culture, 182
  incentives to change, 133, 157
Consultants, 54
Controllable expenses, 59, 182; *see also* Corporate services; Fixed/variable costs
Core staffing schedule, 182
  ensuring appropriate, 17–19
Corporate services, centralization of, 22
Corporate tax, *see* Corporate services
Cost–benefit, 24
Cost centers, 22
  restructuring of during productivity analysis, 36
  see also Fixed/variable costs
Cross-training, 6; *see also* Standards
Customer service, deterioration of, 21

Decision making, emotional, 74–75
Delegation, 62–63
  and accountability, 77
  and authority, 69
  and overspending, avoiding, 73
Disincentives, 3–4; *see also* Incentives

Employees, fixed/variable, *see* specific types

Financial strength, and strategic goals, 95
Fixed employees, 68, 182
  and adjusting standards, 69
  and scheduling, 123–124
Fixed/variable costs, 66–72, 182, 183
  administrative, 67, 182
  administrators and, 67
  departmental managers and, 68–69

departmental composition, 85
measuring, frequency of, 68
splitting, 67–68
step-variable, 70
super-variable, 67
Flexible budgets, 2–3, 182
and productivity standards, 3
Float pools, 19, 182
and productivity analysis, 37
Full-time equivalents (FTEs), 183
and overtime, 14
and registry, 14

Goals, strategic, *see* Strategic goals
Grids, staffing, 177, 178

Historical analysis, 27–28, 128
and skill mix, 8, 9–10
versus benchmarking, 28
Hospitals, performance of large versus
     small, 20–21

Incentives, 3–4, 46, 127, 130–131, 183
to change corporate culture, 133, 154
and consequences, 148–150, 183
executive, 138–141, 141f,
managers, 142–148
     and net operating margin, 140–141
     parity with executive incentives,
          138–139
     "perks," 137–138, 143f
     and social justice, 146–147
     underperformers, weeding out, 144,
          157
mission, linked to, 134–135
outcomes, 131–132
and productivity standards, 137, 147
quality standards, 134–137
and symbolic rewards, 131–132

Labor
composition of in implementing pro-
     ductivity program, 99–100
costs, control over, 66
     agency use, controlling, *see* Registry
     layoffs, 4–5, 5f
     overtime, controlling, *see* Overtime
     skill mix changes in clinical depart-
          ments, 6–10
standards

historical analysis, 27—28
service mix, changing, accounting for,
     59–61, 56f
workload measures, 30–31
Layoffs, and consequences, 4–5, 5f, 22,
     175
versus cross-training, 6

Master staffing schedule, 183
making it work, 120–122
Mergers, in health care systems
cost centers, 20
and cost-cutting, 20
customer service, deterioration of, 21
increased costs, 21
performance of large versus small hospi-
     tals, 20–21, 20f
Micromanagement, 77, 107
Monitoring, 1, 108–109, 118
overcomplexity of, 3, 105–108,
     117–118
and reporting, *see* Reporting
system, 108–109
truncated, 3
volatility/duration rule, 110–112

Net operating margin, 141
Nonprofits, difficulties in productivity
     oversight, 4

On-call workers, 100–101, 183; *see also*
     Fixed/variable costs
Outcomes monitoring, 8, 47, 78
Overhead, *see* Fixed/variable costs
Overtime, 13, 183
analysis, 15f
and fixed departments, 123–124
and float pools, 19
and full-time equivalents (FTEs), 14
and low census days, 15
and low master scheduling, 121
and productivity, 17
and recruitment, 13–14
reduction strategies, 17–18

Pareto principle, 47
Performance reviews, extended, 80
Policy, 152–153
and accountability, 153
committee, 156, 157

and termination procedures, 157–158
compliance with, monitoring, 154–155
principles, 153
tolerance limits, applying, 154–155
Premium labor, *see* Overtime; Registry
Productivity, popular programs, contributing factors to failures of, 2–4, 105, 106

Recruitment, barriers in, 14–15
Registry, 13, 24, 181, 184
analysis, 15t
and fixed departments, 123–124
and float pools, 19
and full-time equivalents (FTEs), 14
and low census days, 14
and low master scheduling, 121
and recruitment, 13–14
role of in implementing productivity program, 100
and training costs, 17
Reporting
analysis, 117, 118f–119f
customizing, 115, 125
format, 113–115
frequency of, 112–113
and monitoring, *see* Monitoring
Responsibility, 184
and accountability, 78–81
consequences of, 85–86, 148
versus the Law of Unintended Consequences, 102–103
Review cycles, *see* Monitoring
Rewards, symbolic, 131–132
Risk assessment, *see* Sensitivity analysis

Schedule, master, *see* Staffing
Sensitivity analysis, 8
Service mix, changing, accounting for, 59–61, 56f
Shareholders, and role in productivity oversight, 4
Skill mix, reengineering, 6–10, 24, 184
and employees, 6–7, 8–9
historical analysis, 8, 9–10
on paper versus in practice, 7–8
results of, 7f
Staffing
approval process, politics of, 75–77
abolishing, 81–83

and extended performance reviews, 80
fixed/variable, *see* Fixed/variable costs
grids, 177, 178
master schedule, 120, 183
adjusting, 122, 170–172
effective, 120, 121–122
low staffing, and registry/overtime, 115
and patients, 121
and testimony, 74–75
Standards
and accountability, 148
adjusting, 73, 89–90
ad hoc program, 93
staffing without, 94–95
development, 83
for fixed departments, 84
becoming "variable," 85
gaining commitment to, 51–53, 54–55, 56–57, 61–62
implementing, 95–101
and consultants, 54
drastic standards, 94
labor, *see* Labor
monitoring, 81, 82, 105
"shaving," 86
for variable departments, 84–85
Step-variable, 70–71
Strategic goals
financial strength, 96
relating to productivity, 95–96

Technology, and management, 106–107
Testimony, 74–75
Turnover, low, 17

Unintended Consequences, Law of, 108–109
Unit of service, *see* Workload measures

Variable departments, standards for, 84–85
Variable employees, *see* Fixed/variable costs
Volatility/duration rule, 110–112

Workload measures, 184
distribution analysis, 99f
for overall organization, 30–31
adjustment factors, 31f